# THE CONSUMER HANDBOOK ON TINNITUS

Richard S. Tyler, PhD, Editor

Auricle Ink Publishers
Sedona Arizona

Libary of Congress Catologing-in-Publication Data

The consumer handbook on tinnitus / Richard S. Tyler, editor.
     p. cm.
   Includes index.
   ISBN 978-0-9661826-7-5
  1. Tinnitus--Handbooks, manuals, etc. 2. Tinnitus--Popular works.
  I. Tyler, Richard S.
RF293.8.C66 2008
617.8--dc22

                            2008001227

First Printing
Printed in the United States of America

ISBN 13: 97809661826-7-5

This book is available at special discounts when ordered in bulk
quantities. Contact the publisher for more information.

Auricle Ink Publishers
PO Box 20607
Sedona AZ 86341
(928) 284-0860
www.hearingproblems.com

# DISCLAIMER

This book is intended for use as a supplement to good medical management of tinnitus. It is not intended as a means for self-diagnosis or treatment. If you are working with a physician, psychiatrist, therapist, audiologist or other healthcare practitioner, this handbook can be very informative about the process you might experience during tinnitus treatment options. The editors, authors, contributors and publisher are not responsible for decisions you or your healthcare team make regarding your diagnosis or treatment for your condition.

No direction, ideas or suggestions from this book should be made or taken without the explicit consent and cooperation of the healthcare individual(s) or team with whom you are working.

# Table of Contents

# CHAPTER ONE

## Overview
## The Consumer Handbook on Tinnitus

### Marc Fagelson, PhD
*East Tennessee State University, Johnson City TN*

---

**Dr. Fagelson** is the Director of Audiology and Interim Chair of the Communicative Disorders Department at East Tennessee State University. Since 2001, he has served as the Director of the Tinnitus Clinic at the James H. Quillen VA Medical Center. Dr. Fagelson's particular interest in the tinnitus clinic centers on the management of combat veterans whose tinnitus is compounded by post-traumatic stress disorder. He received his PhD from the University of Texas at Austin in 1995, MS in Audiology from Teachers College – Columbia University in New York, and BA in English, also from Columbia University.

---

Tinnitus is the sensation of ringing, buzzing, whooshing or other sound in the ears or head without an external stimulus. In short, tinnitus changes people. It can diminish a person's ability to carry out basic life functions, such as sleeping and relaxing. It can influence a person's ability to interact with other people. Aspects of patients' lives once taken for granted and enjoyed can be transformed by tinnitus into negative events to be avoided. Tinnitus patients complain of losing the ability or the desire to maintain relationships. They feel that their identity is changed, and that their value to family, friends, and society is diminished. Patients with tinnitus may find themselves less able or willing to help other people or to seek help on their own. Add to this sense of displacement the fact that tinnitus is not amenable to a simple cure, and the result is a distressing situation for millions of individuals. Despite the lack of a "silver bullet" cure for tinnitus, developments over the past several decades have demonstrated that help is available. Unfortunately, many tinnitus sufferers and many healthcare providers do not access the variety of sources of assistance.

One objective of this book is to provide information regarding the tools available to individuals who need help managing their tinnitus.

Remember, you're not alone, despite the way that the tinnitus may make you feel isolated. In this introductory chapter, we review characteristics of individuals who are at risk for developing and being bothered by tinnitus. We'll also address potential environmental and personal stressors that can worsen tinnitus, how to find and use help for your tinnitus problems, and avenues along which individuals and families who are disrupted by tinnitus can find information and interventions that may improve coping strategies.

Also well worth noting is the use of words that appear in *italics* in this book. All such words are defined for you and appear in the helpful Glossary found just before the Index.

## Who Gets Tinnitus?

Tinnitus affects millions of people around the world. Several long-term health and demographic studies conducted by professionals indicate that approximately 10-15% of the adult population experiences chronic or persistent tinnitus. Nearly half of the people who hear persistent tinnitus are bothered by it, and about one person in 200 believes that the tinnitus substantially affects their life. Tinnitus affects people regardless of race, gender, nationality, and socio-economic standing. Although tinnitus does not always co-occur with a significant hearing loss, tinnitus is more prevalent among individuals with impaired hearing than it is among a normal hearing population (Davis & Amr Rafaie, 2000). However, the correlation between tinnitus annoyance and hearing loss is low (Jakes et al., 1985). You might have a slight to moderate hearing loss, and still be very bothered by your tinnitus.

The results from several surveys indicate that tinnitus can affect anyone at any point in their life. Because males comprise a greater percentage of the veteran and occupationally noise-exposed populations, the trends among younger patient groups indicate tinnitus is experienced more often by males than females. However, when the population sampled exceeds 60 years the gender effect decreases such that prevalence among elderly females is about equal to that of elderly males. The prevalence of tinnitus across other demographic categories shows no specific preference for ethnicity, religion, or socioeconomic status. It is clear that tinnitus is an experience shared by millions, while at the same time it is an isolating and uniquely disturbing sensation. Others might not know you have tinnitus.

Many patients with tinnitus indicate that by increasing their understanding of its causes and its prevalence they can reduce its annoyance. This distinguishes the tinnitus experience from hearing loss or other auditory disorders. So, while it is clear that anyone can develop tinnitus, it may be as likely that individuals annoyed by tinnitus can learn novel coping and management strategies that reduce the amount of distress.

A priority of this book is to provide a variety of useful information. The following chapters are intended to provide a framework within which the reader can find information pertaining to specific causes (physical and emotional) and related problems (such as sleep interruption).

**Chapter 2** addresses causes. It can be useful to distinguish the initial 'cause' of tinnitus, from a "trigger" event, following which an already-present tinnitus becomes worse. Tinnitus can be triggered and exacerbated by a variety of auditory and non-auditory events, and in many cases, the appearance or increase of tinnitus loudness is confusing and frustrating. A substantial number of tinnitus patients attribute the sound to something other than the function of their ears or auditory system. A patient's reaction to their tinnitus depends heavily on their personal experiences, beliefs and psychological state.

Perhaps the most common cause of tinnitus is noise exposure, either long-term or when produced by brief explosive sounds. Other common tinnitus causes include head trauma, whiplash, medications and the aging processes. Often, it is not possible to identify the causes; and there might be several contributing factors that produce a disturbing auditory sensation even when the patient is not affected by an obvious ear disorder.

**Chapter 3** discusses the mechanisms of tinnitus. The precise neural coding of tinnitus within the auditory system and brain is not known. However, it must be linked to spontaneous neural activity, and must be represented in the part of the brain that processes sound. Tinnitus is not a phantom perception; it is real. There is real and measurable neural activity associated with it. It is helpful to think of the auditory system as a complex system of telephone wires. Sometimes the telephone connection to which you're listening gets noisy. A volume control on your phone can help; however turning it up increases the static as well as the signal you're trying to listen to. You can think of tinnitus as 'static' in your nerve fibers. The basic operating properties of the auditory system outlined in this chapter support the idea that the neural equivalent of the unwanted "static" is the tinnitus signal. There are many ways the static can be created, and understanding this helps to appreciate that there are many opportunities to get relief.

**Chapter 4** summarizes the reactions that people experience when they have tinnitus. Although there is no single "profile" for the tinnitus sufferer, many share similar complaints and many endure a variety of additional physical and emotional disorders that exacerbate their tinnitus. Severe tinnitus can provoke feelings of depression, anxiety and anger, and can interfere with basic activities such as sleeping, concentrating, communicating and working.

Tinnitus imposes a sense of loss, the kind of loss we experience when something once taken for granted is taken away. When asked about the bothersome nature of tinnitus, many patients express sadness, frustration and anger that their enjoyment of silence, of peace and quiet, cannot be recovered. The thought of losing silence, or the ability to enjoy silence, may seem abstract to people who don't experience tinnitus. However; such a loss is tangible to an individual who fears they may have to change their lifestyle to accommodate the belligerent and unwanted intruder in their ears and in their head. These emotional responses to the loss of peace and quiet are often, in the patient's opinion, more disturbing than the tinnitus sound on its own.

It is this unique ability to interact with thoughts and emotions that makes tinnitus a particularly disturbing experience that creates in many tinnitus sufferers the sense that they cannot control the tinnitus sound, or that they are losing control of their senses. Patients may attribute to their tinnitus a variety of potentially threatening health and hearing problems. The constancy of tinnitus and the fear it can provoke have the potential to produce a cycle of distress that handicaps the individual across many life activities.

While it is difficult to predict who will be bothered by tinnitus, it is usually easy to tell when someone is suffering from it. Responses from patients regarding their self-assessments of tinnitus handicap reveal that tinnitus severity is most often related to the ways in which tinnitus affects one or more of the patient's basic lifestyle functions and activities. Information related to handicap is often obtained at intake as the clinician tries to understand the causes and depth of the patient's suffering from tinnitus. Studies utilizing patient self-assessments have indicated that tinnitus is most bothersome when it affects sleep, emotional state, concentration, hearing and communication.

Clinicians try to learn about a patient's tinnitus by establishing the ways in which tinnitus affects the patient. Some clinicians may try to quantify the tinnitus sound itself; however it is more important to identify patients at risk for developing emotional responses to tinnitus that exacerbate the problem. A variety of patient intake forms can identify tinnitus-related difficulties as they guide the development of a management strategy. Each person's tinnitus experience has unique qualities based upon their particular auditory and psychological state, as well as their particular lifestyles.

Figure 1-1 contains results drawn from patient reports in several studies and databases showing that the perceived characteristics of tinnitus, its pitch, loudness and quality, result in complaints that can be categorized into functional areas such as sleep problems, communication/hearing difficulties, emotional distress, or impairments related to concentration. These handicaps often influence retionships with friends and family, work and recreational activities. Each person's reaction to tinnitus is unique to their particular perception of

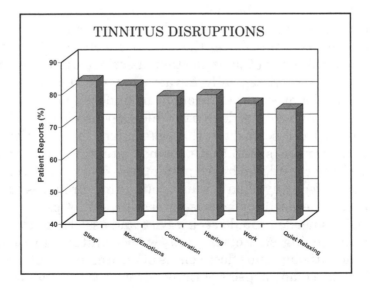

Figure 1-1: Disruptions to daily activities reported by most patients suffering from tinnitus

the sound, and its influence on various life activities. Patients also express concern and fear that the tinnitus sensation will get worse as time goes on. This is usually not the case. But the first few months following tinnitus onset are often full of many fears.

**Chapter 5** reviews some ways people can change the reactions they have to their tinnitus. It is often helpful to separate tinnitus from the reactions to the tinnitus. When tinnitus co-exists with psychological problems the attempt of a clinician to help the patient "divide and conquer" tinnitus from other problems may be helpful, but more difficult to accomplish than when the tinnitus disruption is limited to communication problems. Patients suffering from tinnitus may not attribute immediately their difficulties and distress to a treatable psychological disorder and the clinician may enable a more positive outcome by making an appropriate referral in such cases. Psychological disorders such as depression, suicide ideation, anxiety disorders, and posttraumatic stress disorder are present in more than half of tinnitus patients (Erlandsson, 2000). Patients who experience severe psychological distress related to their tinnitus require services from appropriately trained professionals with expertise in treating such disorders.

One major objective of this book is to demystify the tinnitus experience for patients who seek help from its annoyance. Many people find that learning about a disturbing symptom, such as tinnitus, fosters a sense of control over the condition's effects. Because tinnitus in most cases is not an indication of serious disease or impending deafness, the potentially devastating emotional response to tinnitus can be attenuated through an understanding of tinnitus mechanisms. Indeed, the degree to which a person's life is disrupted by tinnitus is the essential test that determines the condition's severity. A loud tinnitus sound that does not interrupt sleep or concentration will be considered by the patient less severe, and will be dealt with more effectively than a softer sound that produces functional handicaps. The need for help is subjective, and a patient who believes help is needed should seek advice and assistance to learn and implement coping strategies. Help with tinnitus can take many forms, and although the effectiveness of treatment is difficult to predict, there are many aspects of tinnitus distress that can be reduced when the tinnitus causes and effects are more thoroughly understood.

Remember, many individuals with tinnitus misinterpret it as

they believe that the sound they hear cannot be stopped, will always bother them, and may even make them deaf. When it is labeled or evaluated as such by a patient, tinnitus has the potential to be more handicapping than it would be for a patient who recognized that it can be annoying from time to time, but that it poses no substantial threat. One of the more difficult aspects of tinnitus management relates to the observation that two patients hearing a similar tinnitus may respond to it in completely different ways, with different degrees of desperation. For patients to begin the process of learning to cope with tinnitus they must be educated regarding what the tinnitus is, and how it will typically behave under the circumstances in which the patients finds themselves. A priority of this book is to provide that education.

**Chapter 6** puts tinnitus in the context of your life. Each of us is an individual, and none of our lives are without stresses from work and relationships. Therefore, another factor influencing the degree of tinnitus annoyance relates to the patient's surroundings, and the presence of background or environmental sound. Quiet or solitary lifestyles may contribute to tinnitus annoyance when one considers the potential of background sounds to serve as a distraction or masker of the tinnitus sound. Almost 75% of tinnitus patients report that their tinnitus is more noticeable when they're in quiet places and it's even more common for patients to report that their tinnitus makes it difficult to relax. Problems relaxing and maintaining an active lifestyle may inflate the importance of tinnitus to the patient, thereby increasing the priority a patient places on the sensation.

Tinnitus may affect people throughout the day in a variety of environments and circumstances. Take as an example the individual who awakens in a quiet setting and hears bothersome tinnitus. As the day progresses, this person encounters difficulty communicating at home and at work, and upon returning home is once again in a quiet environment. They may not be able to count on a good night's sleep either, thereby perpetuating the cycle of disruption, stress, and fatigue. Tinnitus affects millions of people at their core in this way, where they sleep, where they work and when they try to relax.

Your family and friends often may be reminded that the tinnitus problem is theirs as well. The person with tinnitus may come to rely upon others for support and help that is related to the problems they experience sleeping, concentrating, communicating, and controlling their emotions when trying to cope with tinnitus. For patients to benefit from the support of others, they must be able to explain clearly the ways in which tinnitus affects them and influences their daily routines. Education and practical information regarding the mechanisms by which tinnitus is produced and perpetuated will also help others identify with the problems you experience.

Another objective of this book is to provide you with information that will help you understand your condition, convey the understanding to a support group, and eventually help you cope more effectively with the problem. As patients learn with almost any disturbing or handicapping condition, family and friends can provide emotional support of great value. For tinnitus patients, this support is particularly important because the medical community, in many cases, has little to offer in terms of surefire remedies or interventions. Support of family and friends can counteract the discouragement that many patients experience when they learn that there is no simple cure for the condition. Because primary care physicians and specialists typically cannot treat tinnitus they often pass the patient along to other professionals. What results are feelings of confusion and frustration borne of fear and ignorance regarding the tinnitus and its causes. These emotions can be eased somewhat by a support group that does not question the patient's suffering simply because the patient's tinnitus is neither heard by others, nor validated by standard clinical tests.

A few basic aspects of tinnitus should be prioritized when relating the effects of tinnitus to other individuals. One important point is that most people who do not have bothersome tinnitus hear a tinnitus sound from time to time. These sounds are often described as high-pitched tones in one or both ears that seem to appear out of nowhere, last 30-45 seconds or so, and then disappear. It might be helpful to you if your friends and family could imagine such a sound continuing indefinitely, thereby resembling your experience. When we counsel family members we often point out that the patient's tinnitus is similar to the mysterious transient sounds that most of us hear with some regularity. The fact that such sounds are persistent for the patient can be understood more easily when other people are compelled to use their own experience to imagine the potential problems the tinnitus produces.

Additionally, the need for some patients to have time alone with a hobby, or some activity that they know will reduce tinnitus awareness, must be respected and accommodated even if it takes the patient away from the family on occasion. Perhaps the patient's supporters can participate in such activities, but when sharing the time is not an option the patient's needs should be respected.

**Chapter 7** talks about your hearing system, tinnitus and hearing loss. Indeed, most individuals with tinnitus have some degree of hearing loss in at least one ear. Prevalence of hearing loss in the tinnitus population varies across studies, however, it is typical to find reports that between 75-90% of patients with tinnitus display reduced hearing. Hearing loss that co-occurs with tinnitus may be sudden, unilateral (one ear), and present from mild to profound. Long-term, age-related hearing loss also may be associated with the presence of tinnitus. Hearing loss obviously affects the ease of communication regardless of tinnitus, so it's important that patients understand the effects of hearing loss as it relates to their tinnitus. Even slight hearing loss can impose difficulty understanding certain sounds required for speech understanding. Hearing-impaired people often have difficulty hearing speech in noise, and in more severe cases, also have difficulty localizing sounds. Hearing aids are almost always helpful, but do not restore hearing to normal. As with tinnitus, other family members and friends do not always appreciate the devastating nature of hearing loss. People with hearing loss often withdraw from communication situations, isolating themselves from social environments. Again, in cases when tinnitus is present with hearing loss, hearing aids can help reduce tinnitus annoyance by masking it.

Tinnitus can also interfere with speech perception. People with tinnitus sometimes complain of having to listen to speech "through" their tinnitus. Others confuse birds and telephone ringing with their tinnitus. Tinnitus can limit enjoyment from TV, radio, movies, or other forms of entertainment because understanding conversations and dialogue is difficult and unsatisfying regardless of the patient's hearing sensitivity. Patients may report that speech is not clear or that background noise and tinnitus interfere with the ability to recognize the speech sounds that are vital for understanding. It is important to distinguish the effects of the hearing loss from the effects of the tinnitus. Although tinnitus can contribute to communication problems, many tinnitus patients overlook the fact that some of the same troubles are experienced by people who have hearing loss without tinnitus.

**Chapter 8** discusses sleep, which is one of the most common difficulties associated with tinnitus. The vast majority of patients, regardless of age, gender, and tinnitus characteristics indicate that tinnitus affects the ability to get to sleep, to stay asleep, or to get back to sleep when sleep is disturbed. Andersson et al., (2005) reviewed several studies confirming sleep disorder among tinnitus patients ranged from 71% to 100%. Lack of sleep affects many aspects of a person's life as it induces fatigue and influences psychological state. Several devices are available that can provide appropriate sounds to facilitate sleep (see Chapter 10); however the patient's family may need to appreciate the value of such a device before it is accepted easily. While the patient's supporters may have a hard time understanding tinnitus, they should recognize the effects of sleep loss due to anxiety and the presence of an unwanted distracting sound.

**Chapter 9** discusses concentration difficulties. It's easy to understand how a loud ringing sound in the background could interfere with a person's ability to follow a conversation or concentrate on a required task. Even when tinnitus doesn't affect hearing, its presence can affect the would-be listener by producing an unwanted distraction that influences the ability to keep track of a conversation's topic or nuance. In those cases when tinnitus and hearing loss are present concurrently, the tinnitus distraction can reduce the cues that support communication.

**Chapter 10** reviews the use of sound therapy, including hearing aids and background sound to help tinnitus sufferers. Not all tinnitus sufferers require hearing aids, but those that do often report that hearing aids help their communication and their tinnitus. Having background environmental sound is appreciated by those people with tinnitus who observe that tinnitus is less noticeable when other sounds are present. We often encourage patients to discover on their own the benefits of using sound to interfere with their tinnitus. If a person with tinnitus learns from experience that they get to sleep more easily on rainy nights than on quiet nights, they may capitalize on that observation by using sound generators that mimic nature sounds or small waterfall devices to recreate the comforting sound produced by rain. Others will discover that a fan placed in the bedroom at night provides enough sound to interfere with the tinnitus sufficiently so that getting to sleep is easier than it otherwise would be in total quiet. In those cases when hearing loss is severe enough to make fans or other sounds inaudible, patients may turn to devices with external speakers that can be placed comfortably under their pillow. Many patients find that trying to cope with tinnitus without the use of environmental sound gives new meaning to the term, "suffering in silence."

**Chapter 11** discusses the healthcare professionals who can be helpful in understanding and treating tinnitus. These include audiologists, otologists and psychologists; but some might be referred to others as well. This book is not intended to replace a visit to your healthcare professional. Your tinnitus might be a symptom of some other treatable disease. It is important to appreciate the many professionals who could help you, and what their roles might be. There are many different medical and audiological tests that are available and that might be helpful. In fact, your tinnitus can be measured in much the same way that your hearing would be tested.

**Chapter 12** discusses the variety of medications and dietary supplements that have been used to treat tinnitus. Many individuals report that some drugs and/or supplements have helped them. Unfortunately, at present none are widely accepted as a reliable treatment. Another complicating factor presented by non-prescription supplements is that their composition and uses are not regulated in the US. Manufacturers and retailers of dietary supplements and herbal compounds do not conform to the same Federal Drug Administration guidelines as the prescription drug makers. Therefore, sometimes extravagant claims can be made about their potential to cure or reduce tinnitus without supporting evidence for the claims. Tinnitus also may be an early indication of an adverse reaction to a prescription or over-the-counter medication. If tinnitus develops, then it's important to discuss your use of medications or supplements with a physician.

**Chapter 13** reviews hyperacusis, the experience that moderately intense sounds are perceived as very loud. This is a common observation among some, but not all, tinnitus patients. Patients with hyperacusis often report that they must curtail activities that involve groups of people or noisy areas. At times, they feel the need to withdraw from previously enjoyed places, organizations or entertainment sources in order to maintain a sense of control over their sound environment. Unfortunately, the more a person withdraws from social situations, the harder it becomes to modify that behavior and restore social ties. Hyperacusis often complicates the management of tinnitus as it subjects the patient to a second layer of discomfort. However, there are some emerging treatments. Many hyperacusis patients have reported benefit from listening to low levels of background noise. The use of sound may be counterintuitive because of the aversion the patient has to many sounds. Nevertheless, the use of sound as a therapeutic element can be helpful for some. It might require patience and time, perhaps a period of desensitization, before positive results are realized.

**Chapter 14** provides an overview of the American Tinnitus Association, specifically its roadmap to a cure. The roadmap is particularly fascinating because it allows you to understand the way that researchers think about the problem of tinnitus. It describes in detail, several strategies that show how the mechanism can be discovered, treatments unraveled, tested and refined.

## Conclusions

You might be reading this book for a number of reasons. Perhaps you feel emotionally drained or irritable because of the persistent nature of the tinnitus sound that you hear. You might have difficulty hearing or lay wake at night trying to get to sleep with a cricket sound in your head that won't go away. Or you just can't focus adequately when you're reading because of the ringing. If any of these problems sounds familiar, you are not alone.

It is typical for individuals with tinnitus to search for information on the Internet, in health journals or even glossy magazines found in the grocery store checkout area. Far less typical is the tinnitus sufferer who seeks help from an audiologist or physician. Despite its high prevalence only 7% of the patients followed in a large-scale study contacted a physician for help with the disorder (Davis, 1995). A patient's understanding that there's no simple cure may exacerbate the problem. Because tinnitus is often characterized by the patient as an isolating condition that reinforces the sense that their sensory environment is different from that of their peers, the tinnitus sufferer often searches for solutions or assistance on their own. An Internet search starting from scratch can be helpful, but can also lead to discouraging dead ends and, even worse, suggest false hope in a myriad of 'cures' that carry one guarantee or another. Read this book to deepen your understanding, and equip yourself to ask critical questions of your healthcare provider.

If you're reading this and you don't have tinnitus but rather it is your spouse, other family member or friend who is affected, this book is for you too. Most people who know someone with tinnitus want that person to feel better and to function the way they once did. You can be helpful by understanding and by providing support and encouragement. In this way, the isolating aspects of tinnitus can be minimized, and perhaps some of the emotional strain reduced.

Your search for understanding and relief can start with the pages of this book. But these will not substitute for an evaluation provided by an otologist and audiologist. If you've heard the statement, "There's nothing that can be done about your tinnitus," you're listening to the wrong person. This statement cuts to the heart of why this book was written. The fact that there's no cure yet demands active participation in shaping a strategy, uniquely your own, that helps you experience relief.

## References

Andersson, G., Baguley, D.M., McKenna, L., & McFerran, D. (2005). Tinnitus: A Multidisciplinary Approach. London, England: Whurr Publishers.

Davis A. (1995). Hearing in Adults. London, UK: Whurr Publishers.

Davis, A. & Rafaie, E.A. (2000). Epidemiology of tinnitus; in R. Tyler, (Ed.) Tinnitus Handbook. San Diego, CA: Singular Publishing.

Erlandsson, S. (2000). Psychological aspects of tinnitus; in R. Tyler (Ed.) Tinnitus Handbook. San Diego, CA: Singular Publishing.

Jakes, S.C., Hallam, R.S., Chambers, C., & Hinchcliffe, R. (1985). A factor analytical study of tinnitus complaint behavior. *Audiology*, 24, 195-206.

# CHAPTER TWO

# Causes of Tinnitus

## Paul R. Kileny, PhD

*University of Michigan Medical School, Ann Arbor*

---

**Dr. Kileny** joined the faculty of the University of Michigan Medical School in 1985, and was promoted to the rank of Professor in 1992. He received his Doctorate in Audiology from the University of Iowa in 1978. Professor Kileny has authored over 140 journal articles and book chapters and has lectured extensively nationally and internationally. He is an ASHA Fellow, a founding member of the American Academy of Audiology, and a charter member of its board, a scientific fellow of the American Academy of Otolaryngology—Head and Neck Surgery (AAO—HNS), and a member of the American Otological and Neurotological Societies. He is the recipient of the AAO—HNS Honor Award, of the American Academy of Audiology Career Award in Hearing, and was awarded the Presidential Citation by the American Otological Society in 2006.

---

*Tinnitus* is a common symptom, not a disease. Because tinnitus is the perception of sound, it is closely associated with the hearing system. Thus, there is an anticipation that it is caused by problems and disease processes affecting one or more parts of the ear or the nerve pathways associated with hearing. Indeed various parts of the hearing system are often responsible for the symptom of tinnitus. There are cases where a direct link may be established between some type of hearing problem and the appearance and presence of tinnitus. Other times, there may not be a readily identifiable problem affecting the different components of the hearing system. In some situations, problems affecting other parts of the human organism can also result in tinnitus. This can be important because in some cases when the other ailment is treated, the tinnitus can disappear. However, other times, the tinnitus may persist after the most likely cause has been treated or has resolved.

## General Comments about the Classification of Tinnitus

Tinnitus may be classified in a number of fashions. First, appreciate that just about everyone has experienced a relatively brief perception (10-20 seconds) of a tonal sound. It is sometimes accompanied by a feeling of fullness or slight hearing loss. This can happen once a week, or once every 2-3 months. It is not known if this has any relationship to a more permanent problematic tinnitus.

### Subjective vs. Objective Tinnitus

One of the earliest ways of classifying tinnitus was based on whether or not the clinician could also hear it. *Objective* means that it can be heard by the examiner as well. Patients sometimes report that family members can hear some kind of ticking or pulsing sound emanating from the patient's ear. If one places a stethoscope over the ear or couples it to the ear canal by means of some tubing, or places a small microphone connected to a recorder, then the examiner can in fact hear the same sounds associated with muscle spasm or a vascular problem as the patient does.

*Subjective* means that it is only the patient who can hear the particular sound, and there is no objective measurement available to the clinician to confirm or monitor this symptom. As a result, the nature and severity of the symptom are very specific to each individual. The advantage of thinking about subjective or objective tinnitus relates to possible causes, as objective tinnitus is almost always associated with muscle spasms or vascular problems. Subjective tinnitus is more likely to be associated with inner ear or hearing nerve problems.

Some now prefer to refer to these as middle ear tinnitus or sensorineural tinnitus, analogous to how we refer to hearing loss.

### The Anatomy of Tinnitus

Perhaps a better way of thinking about tinnitus is by which specific anatomical site of the hearing system might cause this symptom. Thus, we may want to consider sites such as the ear canal, the middle ear, inner ear and central auditory pathways. This way of thinking about tinnitus parallels how we think of diagnosing hearing loss. The advantage of this approach to tinnitus is that it may relate better to specific causes and may ultimately relate better to specific treatments.

## Causes of Tinnitus Associated with
## Different Parts of our Hearing System

The hearing system and types of hearing loss are discussed in Chapter 7, and the mechanisms of possible representation of tinnitus in the neural code are found in Chapter 3. Here we discuss tinnitus causes as they relate to different sites along the hearing pathway. However, it should be appreciated that many causes likely affect several parts of the pathway simultaneously. For example, aging likely produces changes in the cochlea and brain. Additionally, although the initiation of tinnitus might be in the cochlea or brainstem, it must eventually make its way up to the brain and be represented there in order to create a sensation of sound (see Chapter 2).

### External Ear

### Earwax or Ear Canal Hairs Touching the Eardrum

One of the presumed causes for tinnitus originating in the ear canal is thought to be the presence of excessive cerumen or earwax. While it's difficult to explain the mechanism of tinnitus caused by excessive earwax, it may very well be that individuals afflicted with this temporary problem may have a heightened sensitivity to normal internal body sounds and may report them as tinnitus. This could be caused by the fact that the excessive amount of cerumen blocks the ear canal, and blocks sounds from the external environment and therefore it is easier to hear normal physiologic sounds such as breathing and the pulsation of blood vessels, all of which most individuals would be unaware of under normal circumstances. Another possible mechanism for tinnitus caused by excessive earwax is if the earwax actually touches the eardrum causing pressure and altering how the eardrum vibrates. Loose hair from the ear canal or specs of skin that naturally peel off may also come into contact with the eardrum, causing temporary tinnitus. In all such cases clearing the ear canal of wax or other debris will provide relief of this symptom (see Chapter 11).

### Middle Ear

Problems affecting the middle ear may also cause tinnitus. These problems can be transient, such as a middle ear infection, which when resolved will result in resolution of tinnitus or other more permanent and serious problems.

## Pulsing Blood Vessels

Pulsatile tinnitus may at times sound like a heartbeat and be completely synchronized with one's pulse. Patients experiencing pulsatile tinnitus describe it as hearing their heartbeat loud and clear in one or both ears. It's easy to verify that this type of pulsatile tinnitus is related to the patient's heartbeat by taking one's own pulse and determining if it coincides with what one hears. Everyone has experienced brief episodes of hearing one's heartbeat perhaps following some type of significant physical exertion but this type of pulsatile tinnitus goes away as one's pulse settles down. Patients complaining of this type of a problem describe it as essentially continuous. They describe that it speeds up when they exercise and that plugging their ear canal can make it sound louder. Some patients are quite perceptive about this problem and will come to the clinic describing that they can in fact diminish the experience of pulsatile tinnitus if they apply pressure to the neck, just below the jaw with their hand or a pillow. Indeed some patients suffering from this problem will tell us that they sleep with a rolled up pillow or towel wedged between their jaw and neck in order to minimize the sound of the pulsatile tinnitus. This type of tinnitus can also be considered *objective*, as the clinician is able to "listen in" using a stethoscope coupled to the ear canal or by using a small microphone connected to audio equipment which also allows a tape recording of this type of tinnitus.

Thus, it's clear that pulsatile tinnitus is somehow related to one's vascular system. The specific cause for pulsatile tinnitus may simply be the presence of very thin bone separating the floor of the middle ear from large vascular structures coursing in the vicinity such as branches of the carotid artery and the jugular vein. At times, however, the presence of pulsatile tinnitus may be an indication of the presence of a vascular tumor referred to as a *paraganglioma* or a *glomus jugulare tumor.* This is actually a vascular anomaly or malformation originating from the jugular vein which can in fact erode the bones surrounding the middle ear and if one examines the ear canal and the eardrum with an otoscope or a microscope one can see the reddish hue of this vascular anomaly as it invades the middle ear. If a glomus tumor is the source of the vascular tinnitus it requires immediate medical and surgical attention (see Chapter 11).

If the pulsatile tinnitus is associated to some lesser malformation or anomaly, first and foremost every effort needs to be made to accurately diagnose the problem and to fully understand its cause. If one determines that the cause of the pulsatile tinnitus is associated with a jugular vein but it's not a glomus tumor, certain types of surgery may be considered. The surgery would involve essentially the blockage of the jugular vein after ascertaining through imaging studies that this was not going to cause a problem with blood draining from cerebral circulation. The principle behind this treatment is to essentially isolate the ear associated with the pulsatile tinnitus from nearby blood flow. The success rate of this type of intervention has received very mixed reviews and typically it's not highly recommended as a treatment for pulsatile tinnitus.

### Infections in the Middle Ear

Patients suffering from middle ear infections often indicate experiencing tinnitus which then disappears following successful treatment of the middle ear infection. This may be associated with the presence of excessive buildup of fluid within the middle ear space, a blockage of the Eustachian tube and this constant pressure might result in the facilitation of hearing of normal physiologic sounds. Another possible cause is pressure exerted by the fluid on the tiny bone chain within the middle ear, which in turn creates a hearing sensation.

### Otosclerosis

This is a condition whereby the last of the three tiny bones in the middle ear becomes fixated within its normal connection into the inner ear thus causing a conductive hearing loss. The tinnitus associated with *otosclerosis* may be due to an increase in the perception of normal internal physiologic sounds or increase of pressure upon the membranes of the inner ear. The disease can also progress into the inner ear causing changes in the bony capsule surrounding the sensitive membranes and fluid-filled spaces that make up the inner ear, and ultimately cause sensory hearing loss which is very often associated with tinnitus.

## Middle Ear Muscle Contractions

An intermittent type tinnitus which may also be objective and doesn't sound like a pulse is most likely associated with the spasm of one of the tiny middle ear muscles. Intermittent tinnitus associated with a muscle spasm may also be referred to as *objective tinnitus,* as mentioned earlier, meaning that it can be heard by the examiner as well by listening to the patient's ear canal.

One cause for such tinnitus may be the spasm of one of two tiny muscles present in the middle ear and attached to one of the tiny bones within the chain previously described. The muscle most often associated with a muscle spasm and intermittent tinnitus is the *stapedius muscle* which shares innervation with the muscles of facial expression. For a variety of reasons this muscle might develop a spasm, and when this happens it initiates a motion of the tiny bones in the middle ear which in turn causes a hearing sensation which is not associated with any external sound. The nature of this muscle spasm makes the tinnitus intermittent and its quality is not tonal at all. Patients suffering from this problem describe the perception of a crackling kind of sound. If one inserts a tiny microphone into the ear canal of these patients for listening purposes, the examiner can in fact hear these sounds as well.

The presence of intermittent, muscle spasm-related tinnitus can also be picked up by other tests audiologists routinely do such as the middle ear *imittance test* and the attempt to record acoustic reflexes. These measurements routinely done in an audiology clinic in particular for a first appointment are sensitive to ear canal volume changes and middle ear space pressure changes and thus can be used to detect the presence of intermittent, muscle spasm-related tinnitus.

## Palatal Myoclonus

This type of tinnitus may also be associated with the spasm of a palatal muscle and if that is the case it is referred to as *palatal myoclonus.* Patients describe intermittent tinnitus associated with muscle spasm as a crackling sound or the sound of paper being crumpled in one's hand. Most patients suffering from this problem can identify certain factors and conditions that trigger this muscle spasm or enhance it. Sometimes it's triggered by swallowing or by voluntary contraction of one's facial muscle. It is of note that while this is unpleasant and at times disruptive, unless associated with some type of neurological disease affecting other muscles in the body, the presence of these muscle spasms has no other health-related consequences. In some ways this phenomenon is similar to a muscle tremor and at times attempts have been made to treat it medically as such. Other solutions that have been considered are surgical solutions consisting of the resection of the muscle responsible for this. All of these attempts at treatment are associated with mixed success (see Chapter 11).

### Inner Ear

Sensory or sensorineural hearing loss may be caused by dysfunction affecting the inner ear and/or hearing nerve and nerve pathways associated with the hearing system. There can be many different reasons and factors that ultimately result in the same type of damage to inner ear structures, commonly the hair cells, as well as other structures responsible for controlling the normal function of the inner ear.

Most of these types of hearing loss may be associated with tinnitus. Damage to the inner ear may be sudden or progressive and the time course of the hearing loss may be also reflected in the appearance of tinnitus as well as changes over time in this symptom. Progressive and permanent sensory hearing loss are caused by almost any factor (for instance aging, *Ménière's disease,* lifelong noise exposure) and will present with continuous tinnitus. The loudness and the specific nature of the tinnitus may fluctuate over time but essentially the symptom is permanent. The specific mechanism of tinnitus caused by sensory hearing loss will be discussed in Chapter 2. However, it is interesting to note that the pitch of the tinnitus often coincides with the area of maximal hearing loss. For instance, patients with Ménière's disease presenting with low frequency sensory hearing loss will often present with low-pitched, at times, roaring tinnitus. Patients presenting with high frequency hearing loss caused by noise or certain medications will on the other hand present with a high-pitched tinnitus. There's obviously a link between the loss of sensory hair cells and the generation of certain types of tinnitus originating in the inner ear.

### Noise Trauma

A main source of inner ear-related tinnitus is excessive noise exposure either associated with work or recreation including the habit of listening to music at excessively high levels. Noise exposure over a lifetime can cause both hearing loss and tinnitus. Often, tinnitus is the first indicator that one was exposed to excessive noise and may be the harbinger of hearing loss that may develop later. For instance, if one shoots a firearm without hearing protection, or if one attends a very high sound level rock concert, sitting in the proximity of a bank of loudspeakers, one may experience tinnitus soon after one of these events. If this is an initial, acute exposure, the tinnitus may last for a few days and if the exposure is not repeated it will eventually subside. If the individual undergoes a hearing test very soon following this exposure, some temporary hearing loss may be documented. Exposures to excessive noise followed by tinnitus may accumulate in such a way as to cause a permanent hearing loss and tinnitus. So in this case, tinnitus may be a welcome and useful warning sign that would help an individual prevent significant hearing loss and permanent tinnitus later on.

## Sudden Hearing Loss

Sudden onset damage may be caused by noise trauma, a physical trauma or certain types of immune system processes. Progressive damage to inner ear structures resulting in a progressive hearing loss may be caused by heredity, prolonged use of certain medications, aging or prolonged noise exposure. The precursor of hearing loss resulting from these various general causes is often tinnitus. For instance, following a sudden noise trauma such as a gunshot very close to the ear without the use of noise protection devices, may immediately result in tinnitus. If a hearing test is carried out soon thereafter, hearing loss may also be detected. If this was a one-time exposure to an otherwise normal ear, full and complete recovery may be accomplished within one to three weeks including the complete disappearance of the tinnitus.

## Medications

The ingestion of excessive doses of certain type of medications such as aspirin for instance can also cause tinnitus initially followed by hearing loss. The mechanism is damage to inner ear hair cells, thus this is another type of inner ear tinnitus. At a certain point in time both hearing loss and tinnitus may be reversible. Medications that can cause hearing loss and/or tinnitus are commonly referred as *ototoxic*. These are medications that may cause tinnitus and hearing loss if used in excess and over a long time. Not all of these medications are prescription medications: aspirin is one of the most common and best known medication-related causes of tinnitus and hearing loss. The excessive consumption of aspirin might initially result in tinnitus. If one then stops using aspirin for a while, the tinnitus will subside. However, if this habit is repeated over and over again eventually the cumulative exposure will cause permanent hearing loss and continuous tinnitus. As is the case with noise exposure, the initial presence of tinnitus is a warning sign that the type and amount of medication an individual takes, places hearing at risk. If this happens you should consult your physician to find alternative medication that does not cause these symptoms. In the past when there were few choices to treat arthritis pain, for instance, the cumulative exposure causing permanent hearing loss and tinnitus was to some extent unavoidable. However, nowadays there are other choices which are much less toxic to the ear. It is important to note that the usually recommended dosage of a daily intake of so called "baby" aspirin (81mg) to avoid coronary disease usually does not result in tinnitus or overall hearing loss risk (see Chapters 11 and 12).

### Ménière's Disease

*Ménière's disease* is characterized by episodic vertigo, fluctuating and ultimately progressing to sensorineural hearing loss, ear fullness/pressure sensation and typically low-pitched tinnitus that may have a tonal or more noise-like quality. While patients with Ménière's disease complain of constant, continuous tinnitus, its nature and severity fluctuate along with the other symptoms of the disease. In some cases an exacerbation of the tinnitus is a predictor of an impending dizzy spell. When the crisis is over patients also report some partial relief of tinnitus. This is an example where the nature of tinnitus coincides with the nature of the hearing loss which also tends to be (at least in the earlier stages of the disease) of a low frequency nature. Within mid crisis, patients describe "roaring" in their affected ear. Any treatment effectively treating the disease may also partially provide relief from tinnitus. A recommendation for a very low sodium diet (<2 gm per day) is often the initial and most conservative treatment attempt for Ménière's disease. If this treatment is overall successful it can also result in some tinnitus relief.

## Aging

It would be very accurate to state that more people over 60 have tinnitus than people between 40 and 60 years of age. From this statement one may conclude that aging equals tinnitus. However, further examination of people over 60 clearly shows that this is a population with a significant percent of people having sensory hearing loss. Since it has been established that sensory hearing loss can cause tinnitus, and that people over 60 have a high likelihood of having this type of hearing loss, then one can easily conclude that the cause for tinnitus in individuals over 60 years of age is the presence of sensory hearing loss and not age per se. Hearing loss associated with aging (also known as presbycusis) is typically sensorineural and progressive in nature. The tinnitus associated with presbycusis is more likely high- than low-pitched and may be reduced when using hearing aids, if necessary.

## Tumors of the Brainstem or Cerobellopontine Angle

Sensorineural hearing loss and tinnitus may also be caused by so-called *brainstem* or *cerobellopontine angle tumors*. These are typically benign in nature and actually originate from one of the balance nerve branches. However, due to their intimate proximity to the hearing nerve they can compress it or the blood supply into the inner ear and cause hearing loss and tinnitus. Often the earliest sign is unilateral hearing loss and/or tinnitus. In most cases in the early stages the hearing loss is of a high frequency nature, and thus the tinnitus described by these patients also tends to be of a high-pitched nature. If the diagnosis is delayed, or if left untreated, the hearing loss can progress from severe to profound and the tinnitus can also exacerbate.

The onset and presence of unilateral tinnitus which may be otherwise unexplained, merits special attention by the audiologist and your physician. Whether associated with hearing loss or not, the presence of unilateral tinnitus may indicate the presence of certain types of disease processes affecting the hearing system. One of those is the presence of an acoustic neuroma (also called *vestibular schwannoma*), which is a benign tumor typically originating from the balance branches of the combined hearing and balance nerve. These tumors may compress the hearing portion of the nerve and this particular mechanical compression may irritate or activate the nerve resulting in the false perception of sound which is tinnitus.

Audiologists and otolaryngologists pay special attention to patients complaining of unilateral tinnitus as it may be the sign for the presence of an acoustic neuroma. Patients presenting with these kinds of complaints typically undergo an elaborate audiological and medical evaluation often times including imaging studies utilized to either diagnose or rule out the presence of an acoustic neuroma. It is of note that while it's possible to have bilateral acoustic neuromas (in particular, patients with *neurofibromatosis II*), most often acoustic neuromas are unilateral.

While these tumors are benign they occupy an area near the brain where if undiagnosed and untreated they could cause various degrees of neurological damage. Therefore a timely diagnosis and intervention are imperative. In these cases the onset of tinnitus associated with the unilateral acoustic neuroma is in a way an advantage as it draws attention to the problem prior to the development of significant hearing loss associated with large tumors.

The treatment for these benign tumors is either surgery or more recently radiation (Chapter 11). If diagnosed early, surgery designed to preserve the hearing nerve and thus hearing may be considered. This can in fact be quite successful with proper patient selection and operative technique. If the tumors are relatively large even with attempted hearing preservation hearing can be lost. Certain operative approaches appropriate for large tumors when there is no useful hearing involve an approach that inherently destroys parts of the inner ear and thus whatever residual hearing there may be is lost. Paradoxically, successful surgical treatment of these tumors with or without hearing preservation often does not reduce tinnitus symptoms.

Thus, patients with complete loss of hearing following acoustic neuroma surgery may continue to experience tinnitus which is completely unchanged in spite of the fact that hearing is completely gone. There are different explanations for this phenomenon. One possible reason for this is that the tinnitus doesn't really originate from the inner ear or the hearing nerve in these cases but from the brainstem itself, and the nerve function patterns caused by the initial presence of the tumor remain after its removal.

## Vascular Loop in the Brainstem

It is thought that pressure of the hearing and balance nerves by otherwise normal intracranial blood vessels that happen to loop and coil near the nerve in such a way as to cause substantial compression may also be associated with tinnitus. This is an area that is some-what debatable, although a small minority of physicians and sur-geons do believe in the association between these blood vessel loops and tinnitus and at times recommend surgery to reposition and iso-late the offending blood vessel in an attempt to alleviate the symp-tom of tinnitus (Chapter 11). There are some reports that indicate that in certain selected cases this may be effective.

## Auditory Cortex of the Brain

It has also been shown that tinnitus can occur without any kind of ear or hearing problems. It's thought that in these cases tinnitus might originate from certain parts of the brain that may be closely associated with the hearing process. One can think of tinnitus caused by inner ear or hearing nerve problems as a bottom up process. In other words, there's some event that has caused damage or changes within peripheral hearing structures activating the hearing path-way in the absence of external sound. In order for sound perception to occur, this information needs to be routed to the brain including the cortex resulting in the perception of tinnitus.

When tinnitus originates from the brain or in particular from the cortex, one might consider this as a top down process since there's no specific participation of any peripheral hearing structures and tin-nitus may be the result of activation of cortical nerve cell patterns identified by the brain as sound. While at times tinnitus associated with auditory cortex dysfunction doesn't have a specific identifiable cause, at other times the general cause can be identified. Among these causes, traumatic head injury caused by some type of blow to the head with or without skull fracture as well as whiplash-type in-jury common in automobile accidents can trigger such symptoms. It's thought that these types of traumatic injury disrupt the normal neural function of the auditory cortex and this may result in tinnitus originating from abnormal neural function in the portion of the brain responsible for hearing. Another source of tinnitus associated with auditory cortex or brain dysfunction may be brain tumors other than the previously discussed acoustic neuroma/vestibular schwannoma.

These tumors may be *meningiomas* originating from the tissue that envelopes the brain, which are benign or malignant tumors as well. These don't necessarily have to originate from the auditory cor-tex to cause tinnitus. As in the previous specific causes, the presence of these tumors might alter the overall pressure exerted on the brain and this in turn may disrupt normal neural function in the auditory portions of the brain. These patterns may be recognized by the brain as sound. Thus, patients with these problems may or may not present with a hearing loss, but they certainly may have tinnitus.

## Non-Auditory Diseases that may Cause Tinnitus

There are a number of conditions which are not directly related to the hearing system that also may be associated with complaints of tinnitus. The exact mechanism of how these conditions affecting other organ systems may cause tinnitus is not entirely understood but there's sufficient evidence confirming association between these conditions and tinnitus.

### Hypertension (High Blood Pressure)

One common condition associated with complaints of ear or head noises is *hypertension* . These patients often describe a pressure sensation in their heads and ears which is at times accompanied by "whooshing" noise. Typically, this head noise is not specifically localized to one ear, seldom has a defined tonal quality, and disappears when blood pressure is effectively lowered by medication. In fact, in some cases one of the initial indicators that blood pressure may be on the rise is the appearance of this type of tinnitus.

### Thyroid Problems

Thyroid problems *(hypo-* or *hyperthyroidism)* may also be accompanied by ear pressure and tinnitus. This is a condition that is caused by either an abnormal increase or a significant deficiency in the production of the thyroid gland hormone. Typically, the tinnitus associated with this condition tends to be of a low-pitched nature and when thyroid hormone production is stabilized through medication the symptom disappears.

### Fibromyalgia/Chronic Pain Syndromes

Patients presenting with chronic pain syndromes such as *fibromyalgia* have a disproportionately high incidence of tinnitus without any specific ear or hearing problems. Fibromyalgia is a chronic condition causing pain, stiffness, and tenderness of the muscles, tendons, and joints. Its cause is currently unknown. Unlike other conditions such as rheumatoid arthritis, there's no tissue inflammation in fibromyalgia. Therefore, despite substantial body pain, patients with fibromyalgia do not develop muscle or joint damage. Fibromyalgia also does not cause damage to internal body organs.

It's often said that tinnitus and chronic pain share some common characteristics. The source of tinnitus that presents in patients with chronic pain is not well understood but the link between these two conditions is quite well established. The nature of tinnitus associated with chronic pain is quite variable.

## Lifestyle Factors that may Cause Tinnitus

### Stress and Fatigue

In general, stress, anxiety and fatigue may either be associated with tinnitus or more likely may contribute to tinnitus becoming more prominent in patients who already present with the symptom. Most patients who suffer from tinnitus will report that at the time of high stress and work or family-related pressures and anxiety will exacerbate an existing tinnitus. While there may be some physiological reasons for tinnitus loudness and annoyance level to increase when stress or anxiety situations present themselves, it's more likely that it is the psychological stress that makes the perception of tinnitus more acute (see Chapter 4).

### Diet and Lack of Exercise

Just like smoking that may cause throat or lung cancer, a high-fat diet and no exercise that may cause blood vessel and heart problems, there are certain lifestyle and environmental factors that can ultimately cause tinnitus. The condition of the tiny blood vessels that feed the inner ear may be affected by fatty deposits and other blockages associated with high cholesterol and sugar. This in turn can impair ability of the inner ear to function properly resulting in hearing loss and tinnitus.

## Foods and Beverages

An additional cause for tinnitus may be food or beverage allergies. These are not as well documented as are noise exposure and ototoxic medications. However, certain clinicians believe that such allergies may be associated with tinnitus. It's difficult to sort through all of these, as in most cases, if allergy tests are actually conducted these turn out to be negative. Additionally, it's not understood how allergies specifically affect the hearing system and cause tinnitus.

## Summary

The causes of tinnitus are many and varied, some of them specifically associated with the ear or the hearing system, others associated with other organ systems or lifestyle issues and habits. Very commonly tinnitus accompanies sensory or neural hearing loss. However, at times it may present as the sole symptom. While most often tinnitus is not associated with serious life-threatening disease, when it appears it needs to be investigated and you are well advised to consult your physician regarding the appearance of tinnitus as a new symptom. When it comes to lifestyle issues or habits, at times changing those may associate with an alleviation of this symptom and at times its complete disappearance. For instance, the reduction of acute noise exposure episodes might ultimately result in the disappearance of tinnitus or at least in the avoidance of permanent tinnitus and hearing loss. In the same manner, the avoidance of the consumption of medications associated with tinnitus will also help this symptom.

It's important to pay attention to the specific causes of tinnitus. Such information will help with diagnosis and ultimately treatment. Researchers are working on different types of treatment modalities, but it's quite clear that one type of treatment will not be effective for all types of tinnitus. For instance, an effective treatment for tinnitus caused by inner ear hair cell damage will not be effective for treatment of tinnitus originating in the brain. It's important to note that as in many other conditions, prevention is essential in the case of tinnitus as well. Thus, avoiding excessive noise exposure, following a good diet and exercise regimen, and avoiding ototoxic medications as much as possible can go a long way in preventing tinnitus.

CHAPTER THREE

# The Neural Mechanisms of Tinnitus

Richard S. Tyler, PhD and Pan Tao, MD, PhD
*University of Iowa*
Anthony T. Cacace, PhD
*Wayne StateUniversity*

**Dr. Tyler** was trained in Audiology and Psychoacoustics at the University of Western Ontario and the University of Iowa. He worked initially at the Institute of Hearing Research in the United Kingdom and is currently a Professor in both the Department of Otolaryngology—Head & Neck Surgery and in the Department of Speech Pathology and Audiology at the University of Iowa. Dr. Tyler has been a visiting scholar in China, South Africa, Australia, Sweden, Poland, Germany and France. He became interested in tinnitus early in his career while working with Professor Ross Coles. His scientific work includes the quantification of tinnitus necessary for its investigation as well as finding different treatments. Dr. Tyler sees tinnitus patients weekly and hosts an annual Tinnitus Treatment Workshop. He has also been the co-principal investigator of a 20-year NIH-funded study of cochlear implants and is particularly interested in binaural hearing.

**Dr. Tao** is currently a visiting research fellow in the Department of Otolaryngology—Head and Neck Surgery, at the University of Iowa. He is a clinical Associate Professor in the Department of Otolaryngology in Peking University Third Hospital in China. After receiving an MD from the Capital Institute of Medicine, he went on to complete a MS in 1998 (which included work in auditory electrophysiology) and a PhD in 2002 both later degrees from the Peking Union Medical College. His research interests are in tinnitus and cochlear implants. He has published more than 10 papers and written two book chapters, which includes work covering a diverse range from measuring the spontaneous discharge of auditory nerve primary fibers examining voice production in prelingual cochlear implant adults.

**Dr. Cacace** is full professor at Wayne State University in Communication Sciences and Disorders. From 2003 to 2007, he served as staff scientist and Associate Professor at the Neurosciences Institute and Advanced Imaging Research Center, Department of Neurology, Albany Medical College. He is chairman elect of the Scientific Advisory Committee of the American Tinnitus Association and is also Editor-in-Chief for the *American Journal of Audiology*. Dr. Cacace has published more than 150 peer-reviewed articles, book chapters and technical papers.

## Introduction

This chapter discusses the possible mechanisms of tinnitus generation at a neural level. Other chapters review tinnitus causes (Chapter 2) and the hearing system (Chapter 7). Chapter 14 discusses a plan for verifying these possible generation sites for purposes of finding a cure. Here, we focus on the possible mechanisms of sensorineural tinnitus.

It is known that many types of hearing loss that begin in the cochlea (that is, those caused by high-level noise exposure) produce tinnitus. For many years it has also been appreciated that the brain must be involved in the coding of tinnitus. There are many causes, many subtypes, and likely, many different mechanisms of tinnitus. One might imagine there might be 100 different mechanisms!

We begin by describing the basic ingredients of how sound is encoded by the nervous system and how this information is transmitted from one nerve to another. We will then describe spontaneous neural activity and sound-evoked activity. Finally, we will speculate with a few examples of how tinnitus might be initiated and coded in these various sites. Actually, we cannot be certain about the mechanisms of tinnitus, but the intent is to give you an appreciation for some of the possible options that are involved.

Some people call tinnitus a "phantom perception" in the sense that an external sound source is not required for its generation. However, tinnitus is not a phantom sound; it is real and real neural mechanisms are involved in coding your tinnitus, just like they are involved with other sounds.

## Transmission Activity of Nerve Fibers

Nerve fibers throughout the body function very similarly. They are constantly active, sending information to and from the brain. Each nerve fiber is like a wire, and many of these wires are placed along channels or cables. Typically, a neuron contains three important parts (see Figure 3-1). A central cell body directs all activities of the neuron. *Dendrites* are short fibers that receive messages from other neurons and relay them to the cell body. Axons are long fibers that transmit messages from the cell body to other neurons. The activity of one nerve fiber is passed on to another at neural junctions

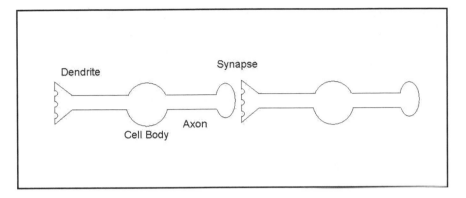

Figure 3-1: The four important parts of a neuron

called *synapses*. The transmission of information along these nerve fibers and across these junctions is determined by chemical reactions. These chemical reactions produce electrical current.

## Action Potentials

Cell membranes along the nerve control and act as a barrier between chemicals on the inside and outside of the nerve. The cell membrane can change the characteristics of the barrier, and when it does, chemicals or ions (notably potassium and calcium) can flow into or out of the nerve fiber. Typically, this begins at one specific place. The chemical reaction at that specific place can affect the cell membrane at the neighboring place. When this happens, the second area changes its barrier properties and starts another chemical reaction. This then affects the next area, and the next, and the next. Thus, a chain of chemical reactions occur along the nerve and the "information" is transmitted. Once the membrane of the fiber changes its barrier characteristics and the chemical reaction occurs, it resets its characteristics back to the normal condition.

These chemical reactions occurring across the nerve fiber membrane create an electrical effect also. The batteries in your cell phone or hearing aid have an electrical potential (a voltage) between the two terminals. This electrical potential is usually 1.5 volts. The electrical potential created across the nerve fiber membrane is only a few millivolts. The chemical reaction is brief at any one place (lasting only about 40 milliseconds). Again, this brief electrical potential moves or 'travels' along the fiber. This brief electrical potential is called an action potential (the voltage represents the potential to transmit electrical activity.) Figure 3-2 shows a simplified picture of an action potential at four points in time as it travels along the nerve fiber.

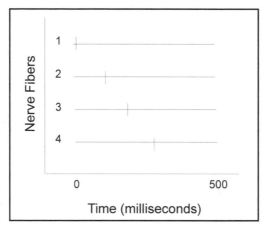

Figure 3-2: Action potential at four points in time

## The Nerve Synapse

To recap what we've learned so far, the action potential travels along a nerve fiber and its job is to tell the next nerve fiber in the sequence that something has happened. But one nerve does not touch the next one. Instead, there's a gap or a small junction between one nerve fiber and the next. The incoming nerve fiber must communicate across the gap to the next nerve fiber. Again this happens through a chemical reaction or a series of reactions. Thus, the communication from one nerve cell to another occurs through the release of chemical substances into the synapse. The "message" is carried by an electrical impulse as it travels or moves down the axon. When it reaches the synapse, it triggers the release of molecules called *neurotransmitters* (see Figure 3-3a). The neurotransmitters flow across the synapse and join receptor sites located on the cell membranes of the adjacent nerve cell (Figure 3-3b).

When sufficient excitatory neurotransmitters have been received in the next neuron, an electrical response is then created in that neuron, and the impulse travels along the next neuron.

After the neurotransmitter is released into the synapse, there are also mechanisms for it to either diffuse away or be destroyed by enzymes so that another reaction can take place.

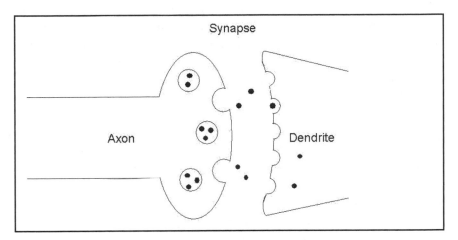

Figure 3-3a: Example of the release of neurotransmitters into the synapse (space)

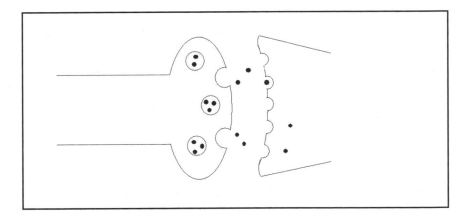

Figure 3-3b: Neurotransmitters flow across the synapse and join receptor sites located on cell membranes of adjacent nerve cell

## Spontaneous Activity

Nerve fibers are active even in the absence of sound. This is because the internal physical or chemical conditions around the nerve or synapse become just right to initiate an action potential. These action potentials, in the absence of an external stimulus, are called *spontaneous activity.* The chemical properties of the nerves and synapses control the spontaneous activity.

In the auditory nerve, normal spontaneous activity varies in different nerve fibers, ranging from less than 1 pulse per second to about 100 pulses per second. There is some indication that neural units with low rates of spontaneous discharge have higher thresholds to acoustic stimuli than units with high spontaneous rates. It is also important to note that spontaneous activity on one nerve fiber is independent (not coordinated with) the spontaneous activity from other nerve fibers. Also, the size or caliber of auditory nerve fibers is also different. Some are large and are *myelinated* (insulation that covers parts of the nerve, minimizing "cross-talk" between the individual nerve fibers); and some are smaller and unmyelinated. Spontaneous neural activity can be different between the large and small nerve fibers.

Nerve fibers in the brainstem are also spontaneously active. There are many junctions, or circuits in the brainstem, and each has different connections to different types of cells that code the auditory stimulus in a different way. Scientists (specifically physiologists) have studied how these nerve fibers code sound and have named them based on their waveform characteristics, like "onset responses," "pausers," "build-up responses," "chopper responses," and so forth. Likewise, the brain and in particular auditory areas of the brain have many interrelated parts. One special attribute of brain activity is that there's some correlation across nerve fibers even without stimulation. It is as if the whole brain is spontaneously pulsing or oscillating at about 1 to 40 times per second or even higher.

## Inhibitory and Excitatory Effects

As it turns out, neural activity on the postsynaptic cell can be either *inhibitory* or *excitatory.* Chemicals that are likely to activate or cause a response on the post-synaptic cell are called excitatory. Chemicals that are likely to reduce or minimize activity on the post-synaptic cell are called inhibitory. The amount of these different (excitatory and inhibitory) neurotransmitters in the synapse determines whether the information from one neuron will be transmitted across the synapse to the other neuron. In the auditory system, excitatory transmitters are glutamate, aspartate, and Norepinephrine. Inhibitory transmitters are glycine and gamma-aminobutyric acid. Of course, it's never quite that simple! Some neurotransmitters can serve as being either excitatory or inhibitory: serotonin, dopamine and acetylcholine are examples. As you will see, if the delicate balance between excitation and inhibition is disturbed, for example, by hearing loss, trauma, certain types of food you eat that contain caffeine (especially chocolate), fluids you drink (coffee, tea, soda) or medications you might be taking (like aspirin), tinnitus can result. The last point is important because it is well known that tinnitus is a side effect of many different types of medications and might also be influenced by the food you eat.

### Efferent and Afferent Auditory Nerve Fibers

The auditory nervous system is composed of two kinds of fibers; afferent fibers that carry information to the central nervous system (brain) and more specifically, from the inner hair cells in the cochlea to the cochlear nucleus. This represents activity from about 90% of all the auditory nerve fibers that come from the inner ear. Efferent fibers carry information from the central nervous system to the cochlea (this accounts for about 10% of the activity). Interestingly, nearly all of the efferent fibers terminate on outer hair cells.

These efferent fibers are thought to have an inhibitory function on the cochlear hair cells, but their entire function is not entirely known. Some researchers think that these efferent inhibitory fibers (sometimes referred to as the *olivocochlear bundle*) might play an important role in the regulation of sound perception (see Chapters 13-14).

### Sound-Activated Neural Activity

Now you know all about action potentials and spontaneous activity occurring in the auditory system even without an external sound. You hear external sounds because external sound causes an abundance of these action potentials in a coordinated fashion. They're initiated in the cochlea and are transmitted to the brain by a series of nerve fibers.

### The Cochlea

The action of the stimulation of the hair cells in the cochlea is described in Chapter 7. The hair cells are the point at which the mechanical movements of the cochlea are converted to electrical action potentials (also known as the *transduction process*). These action potentials are initiated by sound-induced traveling wave motion along the basilar membrane. When a sound stimulates the ear, the *basilar membrane* vibrates and certain hair cells are stimulated. The region of movement along the membrane depends on the frequency of the sound. High frequency sounds vibrate the membrane at the base and low frequency sounds vibrate the membrane at the apex of the cochlea. This motion creates movement and stretching of hair cells, which creates changes in the physical and electrical properties of these cells. At the bottom of the hair cells there are specialized areas where packets of neurotransmitters are stored. In fact, they're tethered or attached to a ribbon-like structure and form a pool of packets waiting to be released. This area is referred to as the *ribbon synapse* and the process of transmitter release is called *exocytosis*.

The junctions at the base of the hair cells are normally spontaneously active, as described above. When the sound intensity presented to the ear is increased, the chemical activity at the base of the hair cells also increases. When there is enough chemical activity, an action potential in the auditory nerve is generated. We also would like to emphasize that the hair cell is very specialized so that the release of transmitters from the ribbon synapse occurs in a graded manner and with great precision. At this stage in processing, this gradation allows for the amount of transmitter release to correspond to the whisper of very soft sound like a child's voice or to the roar of a jet engine. The release also occurs very precisely so our brains can appreciate rapid notes of music from a symphony orchestra or be able to localize sounds in the environment based on subtle time or intensity differences between the two ears.

Inner hair cells release neurotransmitters (usually glutamate) in the junction between the hair cell and the auditory nerve synapse, and the auditory nerve activates or fires. After firing, an auditory nerve fiber cannot fire again until it recuperates (that is, resets itself). This is called the *refractory period* and lasts for about 1 millisecond (one thousandth of a second).

In addition to the inner hair cells, there are also outer hair cells inside the cochlea. Inner hair cells stimulate the auditory nerve in order to pass information on to the brain. Outer hair cells are mostly stimulated by an efferent part of the auditory nerve that brings information down from the brain and brainstem. Efferent activity might influence the mechanical response of the basilar membrane via the outer hair cells, but its role is not entirely understood (also see Chapter 13).

## The Auditory Nerve

The auditory nerve is a bundle of nerve fibers that connects the synapses at the base of the inner hair cells to nerve fibers in the brainstem. Auditory nerve fibers are aligned in an orderly array along the basilar membrane (located at the base of the membranous labyrinth of the cochlea, dividing it into the scala vestibule and scala tympani, that supports the scala media and organ of Corti). Each inner hair cell has about 10 auditory nerve fibers connected to it. Nerve fibers code the frequency of external sounds in at least two ways. First, different fibers respond best to different stimulus frequencies. Second, information about the frequency of the external signal is also present in the time pattern of action potentials. For example, for a 500 Hz tone, many nerve fibers are firing about 500 times per second. For a 1000 Hz tone, many nerve fibers fire at about 1000 times per second. This process, known as *phase-locking*, works up to about 3000 Hz. At higher frequencies, the nerve is not able to follow at this high rate.

As the level of an external sound is increased, the rate of neural firing as well as the number of fibers activated increase. This is how the loudness of an external stimulus is coded. Nerve fibers for hearing are active even <u>without</u> an external stimulus. This spontaneous rate of firing is very likely critical in many types of tinnitus. About 60% of hearing nerve fibers have a high spontaneous rate (greater than 18 spikes per second). There are other fibers that have very low spontaneous rates (lower than 1 spike per second).

Figure 3-4 (top: A) shows an example of spontaneous activity without any external sound. Normally, this spontaneous activity is not heard. Figure 3-4 (middle: B) shows activity produced by a bird chirping. In this example, the nerve is clearly more active and the pattern of activity is much more complex. In fact, it's this pattern of neural activity that is interpreted by the brain as a bird producing its song.

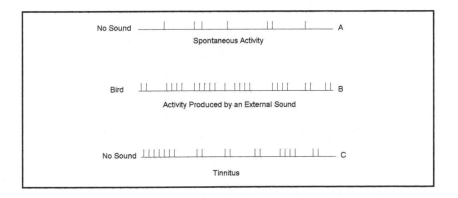

Figure 3-4: Examples of spontaneous activity; A) without any external sound, B) in response to a bird call; and C) tinnitus

## The Brainstem

The auditory nerve carries the action potentials into the brainstem. There are a number of relay stations located at different areas in the brainstem. The main stops, where there are synapses, are the *cochlear nucleus,* the *superior olivary complex,* the *lateral lemniscus,* the i*nferior colliculus,* and *medial geniculate body.* Don't worry about their identification. These are simply anatomical names given to the different relay stations. Of course these structures are found symmetrically on both sides of the brainstem, so there's a right and left cochlear nucleus, and so forth. Figure 3-5 shows a block diagram of the pathways from the cochlea up to the brain. Action potentials from the left ear stimulate the left cochlear nerve, but also stimulate the left and right cochlear nucleus. Similarly, action potentials from the right ear also stimulate the left and right cochlear nucleus. At all relay stations above the cochlear nucleus, there's similar bilateral *innervation,* so that both sides of the brainstem are activated even if only one ear is stimulated.

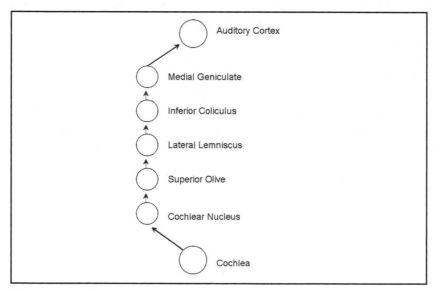

Figure 3-5: Block diagram of the pathways from the cochlea up to the brain

In the superior olive, the minute differences in the timing and levels of the sound from each ear are compared, and this process is thought to be important for determining the direction and location of a sound source. Fibers from the medial geniculate project to both the left and right primary auditory cortex - the hearing part of the brain.

The interactive link between the auditory brainstem and the higher level auditory cortex is demonstrated by the observation that parents will awaken to the sound of a child's cry yet sleep through the sound of a nearby train.

## The Brain

The first stop in the brain is the primary auditory cortex, which is in an area called the *temporal lobe,* located beneath the lateral surface of the head just above your external ear. The primary auditory cortex sends its electrical signals to a nearby secondary auditory cortex, called the auditory association area. It's thought that information processing in these two areas enables us to recognize sounds, words or music.

For most people, the left temporal lobe specializes in understanding and contributes to the production of language. The right temporal lobe is involved in processing sound patterns that become music, or the changes in vocal quality that help to express feelings and emotions. For people who are left-handed or who have experienced damage to the left temporal lobe early in life, language may be controlled by the right side of the brain or by both sides. This specialization of processing within the right and left temporal lobes is probably a matter of emphasis; and more likely than not, both sides of the brain are involved in all forms of hearing.

The auditory cortex is where all auditory information ends up for final processing, interpretation and storage. The complexities of this processing and interpretation are intimidating to contemplate. We are able to identify one individual's voice from thousands of other peoples' voices using subtle frequency differences and at the same time assign the same meaning to a word spoken by an English actor or from a southern stock car driver.

## Possible Mechanisms for Initiating and Coding Tinnitus

We will briefly review several options of the mechanisms of tinnitus. Appropriate citations and a review are found in Tyler (2006).

## The Cochlea

Since the cochlea represents the initial stage of processing where action potentials are generated, and because it is a complex organ with many parts that can become dysfunctional, it's a likely candidate for initiating some forms of tinnitus. Additionally, we know that many changes occur in the cochlea when hearing loss is present.

We will now review several possible mechanisms of tinnitus that might arise from the cochlea.

## Increase in Hair Cell Cilia Motion

Movement of the cilia or hairs at the top of hair cells is thought to initiate the chain of reactions that results in the release of transmitter from the base of the hair cell which in turn initiates action potentials in the auditory nerve. These cilia are normally embedded in a membrane (called the *tectorial membrane*). One hypothesis is that these cilia become disengaged from the membrane and move about on their own resulting in an increased spontaneous activity - and tinnitus.

## Changes in Mechanical or Chemical Properties of the Inner Hair Cell

Another possibility is that there's some abnormality in the inner hair cells. For example, the membranes of the cells might be chemically unstable and therefore could spontaneously transmit information to the bottom of the hair cell; wrongly suggesting that an external signal is present.

## Damage to the Efferent (descending) Auditory Nerve

The role of the efferent nerve fibers carrying information down from the brainstem to the outer hair cells in the cochlea is not entirely understood. Nevertheless, it's possible that a loss of efferent input to the cochlea could serve to modulate inner hair cell function whereby inner hair cells might fire more frequently, resulting in tinnitus.

## Changes in the Hair Cell / Nerve Fiber Junction

Since the action potentials are generated at the synapse between the inner hair cells and the auditory nerve, this area is potentially a primary site suspected for the initiation of tinnitus. For example, there might be an excessive release of neurotransmitters. Alternatively, the capture of the neurotransmitters from the nerve fiber side of the junction might become abnormally efficient. As you can see, numerous options are possible. Increased activity resulting from action potential generated at the base of the hair cells likely contributes to some form of tinnitus.

## The Cochlear Nerve and Brainstem Nerve Membranes

We noted that the cell membranes are directly involved in propagating the action potentials along the nerve. Some changes in the nerve membrane might initiate an action potential, sending information to the brain that might be erroneously interpreted as a sound (tinnitus!).

Back in Figure 3-4, we examined the spontaneous activity of a nerve in quiet (without any external sound being present). Additionally, we examined a nerve that was activated by a bird chirping. Figure 3-4 (bottom) shows an abnormal condition where spontaneous activity is elevated even without any external sound. This might be heard as tinnitus.

We suggested that the spontaneous activity on one nerve fiber is typically independent of the activity on adjacent nerve fibers. Another hypothesis is that a thinning of the protective neural membrane (called the *myelin sheath*) results in crosstalk among closely spaced neurons. This electrical crosstalk is also known as *ephaptic communication.* Thus, when one nerve fiber is sending its action potential along the nerve, an adjacent nerve fiber or nerve fibers, they are also activated. This increase in coherence of the spontaneous activity among different nerve fibers might be interpreted by the brain as an external signal, even when none really exists. Thus, another origin for tinnitus.

## Changes at Synapses throughout the Brainstem

We have emphasized the importance of synapses as a source of tinnitus. There are many complex processes occurring and many opportunities for things to go wrong. As we described above with the hair cell / auditory nerve junction, abnormalities in transmitter release, uptake of the transmitter and restoring the chemical balance to resting states in the brainstem are all potential sources of tinnitus.

Additionally, because the brainstem receives input from many other nerve fibers, there are even more potential tinnitus sources. One of these is when excitatory input from other sources is increased. Another possibility is when there's a decrease, or loss of inhibitory input. We mentioned earlier that some nerve fibers release chemicals into the synapse that decrease activity. If these fibers are turned off or decrease their activity, the resultant output from the synapse might be an increase in activity. As a result, this could be interpreted as tinnitus in the brain.

Another interesting possibility involves the input from other sensory systems that are not normally thought of as being related to hearing. For example, it's known that after complete loss of hearing in one ear, changes in eye position or touch (*cutaneous stimulation*) on the back of the hand can influence tinnitus or for that matter can even turn tinnitus on and off. These phenomena are called *gaze-evoked tinnitus* or *cutaneous-evoked tinnitus.* These types of *somatosensory inputs* (from the body and other sensory systems) can contribute to tinnitus under certain conditions. Although we talked about afferent auditory pathways from the ear to the brain, we should also mention that our descriptions were based entirely on so-called *classical* or *lemniscal pathways.* This is the main path auditory information takes enroute to the brain and it involves primarily auditory input. However, there are also "non-classical or extralemniscal" pathways that respond to auditory, visual, and somatosensory input. Dysfunction in this pathway may also contribute to tinnitus, although mechanisms here are not currently well understood.

## The Brain

Tinnitus can originate in the brain or originate elsewhere and be transmitted to the brain. We believe that there are four broadly defined mechanisms for the representation of tinnitus in the auditory cortex.

First, an increase in the spontaneous discharge rate of nerve fibers in the brain could be responsible for tinnitus. The same mechanisms described above for changes in nerve cell membranes or synapses might be responsible. There are numerous neurons and synapses in the brain, so this is quite plausible. Furthermore, we know that external sounds cause an increase in neural activity in the auditory cortex, so if this were to happen spontaneously, it could easily result in the perception of tinnitus.

Second, tinnitus could be explained by the increase in "synchrony" of spontaneous activity across neural populations. We described this above in terms of adjacent nerve fibers in the auditory nerve and brainstem, and the same factors might play a role in the brain. Additionally, unlike other parts of the auditory system, the brain actually shows some synchrony across nerve fibers throughout. It's like the entire electrical field of the brain is pulsing at about 1-20 times per second. This spontaneous synchrony changes during the cycles of sleep. When an external sound is presented, individual nerve fibers in the brain are active, but this background synchrony continues. Thus, tinnitus might result when local auditory areas of the brain become more synchronized.

Third, there can also be an increase in "bursting behavior," which could be thought of as an altered pattern of spontaneous activity.

Fourth, the response properties of neurons following hearing loss can lead to an over-representation of some frequency regions in the cortex. For example, when there's a hearing loss at 4000 Hz caused by noise exposure, hair cells and auditory nerve fibers that normally respond to 4000 Hz are lost. In the brain, however, the 4000 Hz receptive field area corresponding to 4000 Hz is not lost. Instead, they change their characteristics and respond to adjacent frequencies, like 3000 Hz. However, the nearby fibers that normally responded to 3000 Hz are still present. This reorganization following the loss means that there are twice as many spontaneously active fibers that are sensitive to 3000 Hz. These changes in brain plasticity could be another mechanism for tinnitus.

## Mechanisms of the Reactions to Tinnitus

While we have focused on mechanisms of initiating and maintaining tinnitus, there are other factors that are also important. For example, there are other parts of the central nervous system responsible for the emotional or psychological reactions to various types of stimuli. In the context of our present discussion, regardless of the original source of tinnitus, it is the auditory cortex and associated areas that result in our "hearing" something. However, additional brain areas and systems shape our reaction to what we hear. In fact, whatever the source of our emotional reactions, like seeing something terrible or hearing something frightening, the amygdala, autonomic nervous system and endocrine system can become activated.

### The Autonomic Nervous System

The autonomic nervous system is the part of the peripheral nervous system that acts as a control system for the body, keeping it in a stable and constant condition (also known as *homeostasis*). When a person is in the fight or flight response state, the autonomic nervous system is stimulated and the whole body is prepared for emergency. This will lead to release of adrenaline or other related hormones into the blood stream.

### The Amygdala

The amygdala is a *subcortical* area within our brain that is activated when we have an emotional reaction. The emotional reactions might be initiated by a range of sensory inputs such as sights, sounds, smells, touch or even our thoughts. For example, we might be sad from seeing a picture of a deceased friend or we might hear the screeching of tires that reminds us of an accident we were in last year. Taken together, these events could induce a fear reaction based on a memory, thereby activating the amygdala and setting a cascade of physiologic events into motion. Or we might hear our tinnitus and this might activate an emotional or fear reaction for other reasons. Interestingly, the classic auditory pathways have a connection to the amygdala but it's an indirect one through the auditory association cortex. However, a more direct connection to the amygdala is evident in the non-classical pathways through brainstem connections *(medial geniculate body)*.

### Conclusions

Congratulations! You now know a great deal about some of the very basic ingredients of how we hear, how our brain processes sound, and how our brain reacts to sound. Action potentials, the means of carrying information from the cochlea to the brain, are at the heart of neural activity. These action potentials propagate throughout the auditory system and are particularly influenced by chemical reactions at nerve synapses. There are both excitatory and inhibitory chemicals, as well as neural systems that are meant to increase or decrease neural activity so that a balance is reached.

This complex system of coding and transmitting neural activity is likely at the heart of mechanisms of tinnitus. Therein, we have described several possible tinnitus mechanisms. Your tinnitus is most likely captured by one of these processes or mechanisms. Indeed, your tinnitus is real, it is not a phantom sound! We hope that a better understanding of these mechanisms will eventually lead to a cure (see Chapter 14).

## References

Tyler RS. (2006). Chapter 1: Neurophysiological Models, Psychological Models, and Treatments for Tinnitus. In Tyler RS (Ed.), <u>Tinnitus Treatment: Clinical Protocols</u>. New York: Thieme, pp. 1-22.

# CHAPTER FOUR

# Reactions to Tinnitus

## Soly Erlandsson, PhD
*Professor of Psychology, University West, Sweden*

---

**Dr. Erlandsson** is Professor in Psychology at University West in Sweden. At present she is also Director of the Division of Psychology and Organizational Studies. She became a clinical psychologist at Göteborg University where she received her doctorate in 1990. She had a Post-doc position at Göteborg University 1992-1998. During this time her research dealt with psycho-diagnostic aspects of tinnitus in collaboration with Maj-Liz Persson, MD, psychiatrist and Associate Professor at Karolinska University Hospital, Stockholm. Adolescents' risk-taking behavior and attitudes toward noise and music has become a recent focus of her research.

---

In this chapter the focus is on your reactions toward the tinnitus sound itself, toward the situation that tinnitus creates, and toward other peoples' attitudes and behavior. People's reactions to tinnitus vary widely from one individual to another. The different topics in this chapter are meant to give you a diversified impression of the various distressing aspects that tinnitus can trigger:

- grief over the loss of silence
- emotional upset and panic
- preoccupation with harmful sounds
- tinnitus and sleep disturbance
- weak and vulnerable feelings
- fear of losing your mind
- guilt
- adjustment to the sound
- a need to share your experiences with others
- using metaphors (the pearl and the oyster)

### Grief over Loss of Silence

In many instances tinnitus onset can give rise to fear that the sound is going to be permanent, meaning that you will never again experience silence. As human beings, we have different needs, and when some of these most important needs cannot be met, we simply do not feel very well. The onset of tinnitus is especially stressful to people who love to be in silent places because it gives them time to reflect and think about things that are of vital importance to them. In this chapter, I will focus on peoples' reactions after the onset of tinnitus. It's important to emphasize that negative reactions in most instances subside after a few months or a year or so. Reasons for prolonged negative reactions are unknown and also vary across individuals. It might be related to the cause of tinnitus (for example, a noise trauma or chronic disease that influences many aspects of a person's life).

There are many different situations and conditions that can give rise to sorrow when you suddenly experience a loss of hearing or onset of tinnitus or become extremely sensitive to loud sounds. To become hearing impaired is an example of a situation that involves all aspects of life; you as an individual, the members of your family, work, and leisure time. In the same way, tinnitus can cause both acute and prolonged problems at different levels of social life. Considering this, not only must you be given an opportunity to express grief over the loss of silence, but also be able to grieve that you no longer feel engaged in your work as you used to, or that you cannot enjoy meeting your friends as before. Life is not what it used to be, and when you look back on the situations you enjoyed most, you realize that these situations are now more distressing than joyful.

Interviews with patients for whom tinnitus has been a severe problem have made it clear to me that tinnitus also can deprive someone of her or his freedom (Erlandsson, 2000a). This statement is an example: "My irritation concerned the fact that in many ways, I was deprived of my freedom, that there were things that I couldn't do. For example, I couldn't play the guitar."

What does it mean to lose one's freedom? Usually we talk about freedom as something we experience in a democratic political system where we have the freedom to speak and write. But freedom can also mean being able to act and do things spontaneously in a non-reflective way. It can be the most natural thing for me to take my guitar and play, if I like to do so. But when music can make me worry about possible negative effects on tinnitus, I can no longer enjoy playing the guitar. It's not a spontaneous act anymore.

There are many examples of restrictions in peoples' freedom of actions when tinnitus occurs. You might have to avoid certain situations and become limited for a number of reasons due to the noise in your ears. In young people, tinnitus can hamper their future plans. A young woman worries about her education and how to manage her studies due to the annoying sound in her ear. A young man is afraid that his future plans to become a professional musician cannot be fulfilled. To be plagued both by tinnitus and dizziness can also interfere with a woman's desire to have a child. For a period of time, I saw a patient who had Ménière's disease and was very ambivalent about being a mother because of her tinnitus, dizziness and hearing loss. However, she eventually decided that not having a child would mean that she had let the tinnitus decide her future. She took control of her life and became a confident and responsible mother, a more appropriate and satisfying situation.

The loss of silence can have an impact on people for a long time. Normally, when we lose something there's a period of grieving, which is often appropriate and helpful. It can be hard for a person with tinnitus to grieve because he or she does not feel that it is correct to mourn the loss of silence. The sorrow is often ignored by professionals who are most concerned with how the patient's problem should be managed within a healthcare regime. One role of the professional would, therefore, be to create an atmosphere where such a grief process can take place. We must remember that it's normal to grieve over things we've lost in life. The grief for silence or hearing loss is very similar to grief for the loss of a loved one. Some people can manage to grieve over their loss by themselves while others need comfort and help in order to go through this process. There are, however, very few rituals, if any, to help us manage a loss that occurs when someone becomes hearing impaired or acquires tinnitus. You should feel free to discuss this loss. Tinnitus is an unrecognized affliction and is not apparent to anyone else.

## Emotional Upset and Panic

It can be a strange feeling to find yourself becoming emotionally unstable and panic-stricken after the onset of tinnitus. The most frightening thought for someone who suddenly starts to hear a strange sound inside the ear is that it never will disappear. In interviews patients have described their alarming thoughts following the debut of tinnitus: "A tremendous fear. That's what I remember. I was terribly afraid that it would become permanent." From one day to the next, you can become a fragile and worried person with no former knowledge to help you understand the situation. You might think that it's impossible to cure tinnitus, as it is with other conditions like headaches or back pain. It is also said by many professionals that you have to learn to live with the noises without providing any guidance. So the panic has a logical ground! I would say that it's normal to react with some degree of "panic" with an acute tinnitus because there are most often no cures available at first. In fact, many people are convinced that there's nothing that can be done. You can sometimes sense from professionals that it would be a disaster for them if they were to get tinnitus. These attitudes from society do not enhance the probability of someone being prepared to cope with tinnitus when it first appears. One tinnitus patient gave voice to such a preconception: "I was paralyzed with terror....I knew that something terrible had happened to me."

Tinnitus seems to be linked to anxiety in various ways. Young people who react with strong fears when tinnitus occurs describe their panic attacks as more frightening and more difficult to cope with than the tinnitus sound itself. Panic can, for example, appear after long-term stress in many life circumstances, even without tinnitus or hearing loss. This can also be seen as a positive observation, since a decrease in the general stress in one's life typically reduces the stress associated with tinnitus.

In meeting with patients who seek help, the clinician might learn from a client that there has been a history of severe stress and tension before the onset of tinnitus (Erlandsson, 1998). Recently, a young woman described how she was suddenly afflicted with tinnitus and became extremely upset and panic-stricken. Without warning, she heard a high-pitched noise in one ear and believed at first that it was an external sound coming from somewhere in the apartment. The sound didn't go away. She was convinced that the onset of tinnitus was related to her current life situation in which a number of sad episodes in her family had taken place. Both her father and her mother had become seriously ill at the same time as she was breaking up a relationship with a boyfriend of seven years. It helped her to handle the panic when she realized that she had been under an unusual amount of stress and that tinnitus seemed to be the reaction. Another client told me that he noticed his ears felt blocked and the buzzing sound came after a stressful day. Someone who is experiencing an increased and prolonged level of distress can have little tolerance for even a faint sound in the ear or head.

Another problem arises because it's not always easy to identify the cause or source of the tinnitus. Patients might seek help for tinnitus which they believe is a symptom entirely related to a defect in the ear. When the clinician can't identify any defect in this organ, the client doesn't know what to do and what to believe. To whom shall you turn if nothing is wrong with the ear? One voice reflected this dilemma: "I think it's hopeless to have tinnitus, that's all. I must learn to accept it. If I could choose, I would like them to cut that piece off, but there's nothing that is physiologically wrong, they say."

Many healthcare professionals are not prepared to give the client a view other than the biological one. To be able to understand the way the psychology and the body are intertwined, there's a need for a humanistic approach. We must understand that suffering is often more related to our life situation in a psychological sense than to our physical body. Examining the psychological aspect of tinnitus as suffering requires an appreciation based on understanding of peoples' narratives about their own experiences (Tyler & Erlandsson, 2002).

## Preoccupation with Bothersome Sounds

It is not unusual that people are bothered or annoyed by certain sounds in their surroundings, especially those sounds that they can't control. Someone who is very concerned with the sound environment and how to control it might react more intensely and fearfully to the onset of tinnitus than someone who pays very little attention to everyday background sound and noise. Annoyance to sounds can also appear as a consequence of a hearing deficiency. This sometimes results in the person being particularly annoyed by sounds of certain frequencies. In such instances, it's likely that tinnitus is experienced as more annoying if the frequency of the external sound is in the same frequency range as the tinnitus. It can be difficult for a person with a sound annoyance problem to habituate (get used) to the tinnitus (see Chapter 13).

What is it that makes people become annoyed to sound? In most instances, there's no physical sign to explain this annoyance. One interpretation that seems particularly important is the level of arousal that influences the way people react to stimuli. High arousal (after prolonged stress) makes it more difficult to get used to a sound, and this is especially true if the sound is perceived as harmful. Tinnitus might be perceived as something harmful because you can't imagine how you're going to live with it. Figure 4-1 depicts this negative cycle. For example, tinnitus occurs after a period during which you have been under a high level of stress (Erlandsson, 1998). Your reactions toward the tinnitus become strongly negative as the situation makes you upset and worried. Thereby you perceive that tinnitus is getting louder (escalating) which increases the level of arousal and the vicious cycle has developed.

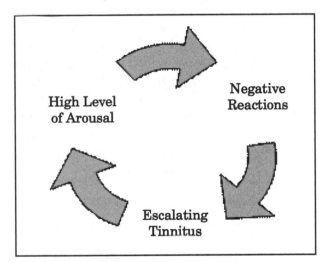

Figure 4-1: The negative reinforcing cycle between tinnitus and your reactions to it

We sometimes refer to people as extraverts or introverts. These concepts are part of a theoretical framework in psychology. Originally, characteristics of introverts and extraverts were described by the psychiatrist and psychoanalyst Carl Gustav Jung as two different attitudes. Jung presented his theory on personality types the first time in 1921 (Jung, 1921). A person who is an extravert feels confident with new and unknown things, can easily adapt to a given situation and is influenced by objects and events in the external world. The introverted person shows a keen interest in his or her own psyche, and the external world is not the focus of attention. There are no pure personality types as introverts and extraverts, but rather a tendency toward one or the other. We can speculate about what Jung's theory on the introvert/extravert personality type adds to the understanding of adjustment and the process of habituation to tinnitus. Is it, for example, easier for someone with a more extraverted attitude to adjust to a new tinnitus than someone who has a more introverted attitude to life?

Tinnitus is sometimes experienced as impeding the ability to hear in some listening situations. When the attention is directed inward on the tinnitus sound, and not toward the outside world, it can be difficult to concentrate and listen to what people say. If you're absorbed by worrying thoughts about the situation and how to deal with it, it's natural that your interest in others diminishes. By listening to tinnitus, you might feel that you get an illusionary control over the sound. It can then be acknowledged as a physical symptom which is more acceptable than something psychologically uncontrolled.

## Tinnitus and Sleep Disturbance

Many problems that we have to deal with through life can be draining and give rise to heightening levels of stress and, as a consequence, insomnia. Sleep disturbances influence the way you handle your daily routine, work and communication with others. Disturbed sleep, fatigue and loss of interest in your favorite things in life are examples of what patients describe as negative factors related to their tinnitus. Even children who complain of tinnitus are often found to suffer from sleep problems. McKenna (2000) reported that sleep disturbance is one of the most common complaints associated with tinnitus in about half of his study group. He suggests that it would be more helpful if a complete assessment of sleep complaints would be used. For example, someone with tinnitus and severe sleep problems should benefit from attending a sleep clinic. This usually includes a detailed interview, diary records of sleep behavior, and recordings of breathing and brain activity during sleep. With all these measurements, it's possible to get an accurate view of sleep difficulties associated with tinnitus and to plan treatment.

To be exhausted after long nights without enough sleep can cause health problems, and there can be a secondary risk for a person suffering from insomnia to develop mental health problems. Sleep disturbances have, for example, been identified in mood and anxiety disorders, panic disorders and in alcoholism. Quality of sleep seems to be relatively independent of social factors such as gender, social class, education, marital status, and religion. Not even social support is found to be of any relevance for the occurrence of sleep problems. Whether or not tinnitus is the cause of a person's sleep disturbances can be difficult to sort out. It might be hard to believe, but there are also examples of positive effects of tinnitus on sleep. One client reported that tinnitus was as good as a sleeping pill because the sound made him relaxed so that he more easily could fall asleep at night.

## Weak and Vulnerable Feelings

Emotional reactions associated with severe tinnitus vary across individuals, and can include being easily disturbed, annoyed, anxious, depressed, ambivalent, feeling uninvolved and worthless. Reactions like these might lead to feelings of being a stranger to yourself. This can be a scary experience, making it difficult to maintain self-confidence and a desperate hope that things will improve. One patient put it this way: "When my tinnitus started, it was like a complete change of identity." Participation in common activities can also become very restrictive. One client discussed the fact that she was unable to understand the reason for her emotional irritation and anger: "It's difficult to know what is due to tinnitus and what is due to other things in my life. As you get older, maybe you react more strongly than in earlier years. I'm so much more active now than when I was young, so maybe that's why I have tinnitus. As you become older your reactions might be stronger than before, but I don't know if these reactions are due to tinnitus or due to me becoming older."

Feeling that tinnitus has a negative influence on the person's zest for life is exemplified by a loss of enthusiasm for small things in day-to-day living. Mood variations also seem to be a common experience accompanying tinnitus complaints. One woman described this: "Tinnitus makes me very depressed during certain periods and it takes almost all the energy I have. I need all my energy to keep myself going and to function at work."

The immediate reaction when something unexpected and fearful happens is that we feel anxious and vulnerable. Anxiety and worrying thoughts make it difficult to concentrate and can interfere with our work. When concentrating on a challenging task, you might feel distracted by tinnitus and, as a consequence, cannot get your work completed.

## Fear of Losing Your Mind

Tinnitus encroaches on personal integrity, perhaps partly by its location in the head where intellectual and mental capacity also occur. Tinnitus is a discomfited sound that you want to ignore, but which the psyche somehow 'forces' you to pay attention to. To concentrate on the sound can be a way to establish a necessary inner balance in order to avoid psychological turmoil. Secondarily, relationships with others are entangled by the fact that it's difficult to share with someone who does not have the same experience that living with tinnitus is an undesirable inner sound. This was expressed by another client: "No one can understand how it feels to be forced to listen to this noise day and night." The latent message might be: "No one understands how I suffer" - and implicitly - "no one understands me!" (Erlandsson, 2000a). Tinnitus, symbolically viewed, can create a wall between the person and his or her social environment. This "invisible wall" can confirm the experience of not being understood and increase the fear of failure in social relationships.

Interviews with patients with tinnitus have highlighted a symbolic distinction between the physical body as something distinguished from the self (Haak, 1997). In such expressions, the body is described as "somebody that speaks to the self" - the body and the self are involved in a dialogue. Words such as "weakness," "splitting" and "bodily eruption" are often found in the interview material. Tinnitus is perceived as the cause behind both bodily and mental splitting and fear of being overwhelmed by the sound. You could think of this as an example of a person who is psychologically vulnerable and who reacts in a fearful manner by the influence of his or her defense mechanisms. Severe tinnitus suffering might in some cases exacerbate symptoms that are related to mental health (Erlandsson & Persson, 2006).

Explanations for why tinnitus turns into a chronic handicap for some can be found in psychological theories on personality and individual development which is significant for the understanding of vulnerability and suffering. You could be vulnerable due to experienced life stress, anxiety or a depressive disorder. People who've been traumatized by war or severe accidents can also be vulnerable because they suffer from post-traumatic stress disorder. But also social factors, like emotional support, compassion and the quality of the encounters with professionals and caregivers are of considerable importance. A problem that limits a person's ability to live a "normal life" and gives rise to severe anxiety and depression secondarily, although there is no serious illness involved, conveys an important psychological message. The reason for the individual to seek help can be strong panic, not over a feared physical disorder, but rather a fear of not being able to mentally control tinnitus and as a consequence suffering a mental breakdown. In meeting with someone who is afraid of becoming mentally ill, the professional must take the time it takes for the patient to be able to talk about these fears.

## Guilt

Feelings of guilt toward family and friends for being easily upset and sometimes angry increase the burden. There are many examples of situations where people feel guilty because they cannot live up to what they themselves see as their "normal" behavior, i.e., the way they used to be. Guilt feelings arise when a partner in a relationship cannot live up to expectations due to the handicapping effects of tinnitus. One patient described that she felt sorry for her husband because she was unable to enjoy life as a pensioner and was not able to accompany him on trips abroad that they both had looked forward to. It's not unusual for someone with tinnitus to emphasize how extraordinary their partner is, which is in great contrast to how badly one experiences one's own behavior in the relationship. And this is also a basis for guilt feelings: "How can you be so patient and nice to such an awkward person as me?" In this way the relationship can be unequal, as the needing person becomes unnaturally dependent on his or her partner. It is important to be aware of how roles in the relationship can change and become unequal due to a partner's impairment. A good solution to the problem is to be open about it. In that way you can understand the dynamic within a relationship and how a handicap can change the balance between two people who are dependent on each other.

In addition, relatives sometimes have feelings of guilt because of their sense of helplessness—feeling that there's not much that can be done in this situation for their family member. Many people believe that tinnitus is a chronic condition and that it's very hard to live with it. If this is the way you think, the likelihood that you will be able to comfort your parent or spouse who complains of tinnitus is indeed very low. We must believe that tinnitus can be dealt with and that there's hope for improvements. You can show an empathic understanding of the way your ailing friend or relative reacts, but also communicate your hope that improvements are to be expected in the near future. We refer to this as being a "deputy" hope for someone during a difficult period in life.

## Adjustment to the Sound

A significant word, often used when someone has a deficiency or a chronic illness, is the term "adjustment." Some people even use the word acceptance, since they think that you must accept the deficiency in order to take a step forward in the adaptation process. The practitioner might say that you have to adjust to the hearing loss or tinnitus. For some people, to adjust (or accept) is the same as giving up. For example, I must adjust to the situation that pain is part of the disease or that tinnitus is a plague all day. Then I might as well give up my ambitions to get well, since I cannot really imagine being well. If you adjust to the situation of having tinnitus, you might not see that things are changing; for example, that your tinnitus actually has become less intrusive the last couple of months.

"Tolerance" seems to be a better choice of a word since it is more neutral. You should be able to tolerate that you've got tinnitus even if it's not something you wish to have. We speak about level of tolerance and that such a level is individually shaped, but also dependent on the situation (context). We can be tolerant in one situation and not in another. I can be tolerant toward noise in general, but when I'm perhaps tired or feel distressed, the tolerance fades away. It's the same with tinnitus and tolerance. When things are going your way and you feel somewhat relaxed, your tinnitus could seem a rather minor problem. But when you're under heavy stress with tension in your body, tinnitus can become a major trouble. If you're able to see that the level of annoyance is related to your emotions and stress reactions in a given situation, you could also find it easier to tolerate having tinnitus.

## A Need to Share Your Experiences with Others

We used to say that a shared burden is half as heavy to carry and a joy that is shared is a joy made double. As professionals, we often learn from clients that sharing the difficult experiences with others can ease one's mind and make the situation more tolerable. A group of clients who see that talking to others can be a cure is moving forward by sharing their thoughts in a therapeutic way. Group members are valuable for each other in many different ways. Emotional pain is difficult to express to someone outside the group, but in a group setting where people are interested in each other's various experiences, this can also be articulated. Not everyone has the courage to show others a "weak" and vulnerable side of oneself. This can especially be difficult for men, as the ideal masculine role is considered to be invulnerable and self-assertive. Here the group can make a difference, and the way the participants confide in each other can increase the openness among them—including the men.

Even if someone is longing for companionship it can be hard to fulfill this need since there's not much energy left over for social life. To go to a friend's party can be experienced as a strain, yet having a circle of close friends is necessary for most people. In studies where I examined perceived social support given by family and friends, it was clear that support from a relative was not enough for the decrease of handicap due to tinnitus. Perceived social support by a close relative was more frequent in the male patients with tinnitus, but it did not have a pronounced positive influence on the perceived handicap. There are many examples in research other than tinnitus studies, that a social network is the best social support, indicating that relatives, friends and workmates are there for you when you need them.

## Using Metaphors

When working with clients who were worried because they didn't know how they should learn to live in harmony with their tinnitus, I tried to find the right words or metaphors that could be useful for them. You can't just say to someone, "you have to learn to live with the noises," because this is just what the client has tried and not been able to do and the reason for him or her to consult a specialist. Practitioners have to be sensitive enough and to give their clients tools that they can use for such a learning process. With time, experience, patience and understanding, your level of tolerance will increase.

Next is an example of a metaphor that I used while working with clients with tinnitus in group psychotherapy. It's an example of the power we actually have if only the fears can be defeated.

## The Pearl and the Oyster

Tinnitus can create anxiety and disturb balance in humans, but this is not a "law of nature." We find an example of an organism, the pearl oyster, which protects itself against a grain of sand by producing a shelter that shares the characteristics of the oyster shell. The grain of sand is able to accommodate to the milieu of the inside of the oyster. This process is necessary for the production of beautiful pearls, but it's also an example of a process of adaptation that can be found in nature. The oyster does not know about the process itself, but nevertheless it contributes to change and to the refinement of the grain of sand. Adaptation is an essential phenomenon in nature. Likewise, human beings' survival and mental health is strongly related to the process of adaptation and normalization.

By analogy with the oyster's production of the "pearl," which implies a form of neutralization instead of expelling the strange object, the mind can seek to balance the tinnitus sound to get it under control instead of fighting against it. For example, I can try to influence the negative experience by imagining that the noise in my ear is coming from the rushing of the sea or the spring creek in the woods. Sounds coming from natural sources like water, sea and wind are something that we most often associate with relaxation and positive experiences while all the undesirable noises people are exposed to make them vigilant and tense. By using the power of thought over what is experienced as destructive, "the grain of sand can become a valuable pearl.

(Soly Erlandsson, 2000b)

## References

Erlandsson, SI. (1998). Psychological counselling in the medical setting: some clinical examples given by patients with tinnitus and Ménière's disease. *International Journal of Advanced Counselling,* 20: 265-276.

Erlandsson, S.I. (2000a). Pychological profiles of tinnitus patients. In: Tyler, RS (Ed.). Handbook on Tinnitus. San Diego, CA: Singular Publishing Co, pp.25-58.

Erlandsson, SI. (2000b). Tinnitus: ljud som bärare av psykisk smärta – empiriska och teroretiska perspektiv (Tinnitus: sounds carrying psyclogical pain – empirical and theoretical perspectives). In: Carlsson, SG., Hjelmquist, E. & Lundberg, I. (Eds.). Delaktig eller utanför. (Participate or being outside). Boréa Bokförlag, pp. 571-578.

Erlandsson, SI. & Persson, M-L. (2006). A longitudinal study investigating the contribution of mental illness in chronic tinnitus patients. *Audiological Medicine,* 4: 124-133.

Haak, M. (1997). Bilder av tinnitus - en kvalitativ studie om att leva med tinnitus (Images of tinnitus – a qualitative study on how to live with tinnitus). Department of Social Work, Göteborg University.

Jung, CG. (1921). Psychologishe Typen. Zurich: Rascher Verlag.

McKenna, L. (2000). Tinnitus and insomnia. In: Tinnitus Handbook, Tyler, R. (Ed.). Clifton Park, NY: Singular Thomson Learning, pp. 59-84.

Tyler, RS. & Erlandsson, SI. (2002). Management of the tinnitus patient. In: Luxon, LM., Furman, JM. Martini, A. & Stephens, D. (Eds.). Textbook of Audiological Medicine, Oxford, England: Isis Publications, pp. 571-578.

## CHAPTER FIVE

# Changing Reactions

### Laurence McKenna, PhD

*Royal National Throat, Nose & Ear Hospital, London*

### Gerhard Andersson, PhD

*Linköping University and Karolinska Institutet, Sweden*

---

**Dr. McKenna** has worked as a clinical psychologist at the Royal National Throat Nose & Ear Hospital for the past 24 years. During this time he has been involved in the study of tinnitus and other audiological disorders and in the psychological management of patients with these problems. He is head of the team of psychologists working in Adult Audiological Medicine and is a member of the cochlea implant team. Other work at Guy's and St Thomas' Hospitals in London has included the assessment and management of patients with neurological disorders, medico-legal work, management of attempted suicide patients, cochlea implantation and sleep disorders. He is an honorary lecturer at the Ear Institute (UCL) and Visiting Fellow at the University of Bristol.

**Dr. Andersson** is professor of clinical psychology at Linköping University, Sweden. He is also guest professor at the Karolinska Institutet, Sweden. Apart from his research he also spends his time as a clinician working with tinnitus patients. Professor Andersson has done research and published papers on various aspects of tinnitus, including cognitive behavioral therapy, cognitive processes, brain imaging and personality. He is also the author of three books about tinnitus. Professor Andersson often lectures about tinnitus and advocates a multidisciplinary approach to its treatment. Probably his most important contribution to the field is development of In ternet- delivered treatment of tinnitus distress.

---

## Introduction

This chapter describes the ways in which people react to tinnitus and how these reactions come about. Reactions to tinnitus are understood within a cognitive behavior therapy framework. How a person thinks about tinnitus is seen as the most important thing. How we think about tinnitus can be influenced by things such as our stress level which can lead to overly negative or "middle of the night" thinking. This thinking can lead to changes in our behavior that may reduce anxiety in the short term but keep the problem going in the long term. We discuss ways of identifying and changing these thoughts and behaviors. When a person is successful in changing from "middle of the night" thinking to a more balanced perspective, then tinnitus becomes less intrusive.

Our approach to understanding tinnitus and people's reactions to it is based on cognitive behavior therapy (CBT). This is a psychological approach that takes account of the links between the physical aspects of tinnitus and the emotional reactions to it. There is strong research evidence that this approach helps people with tinnitus and with many other problems.

### What Type of Reactions do People have to Tinnitus?

The first really important thing to know about tinnitus is just how many people have it. Ten per cent of the adult population has tinnitus. This is a huge number of people. The next thing to know is that there's a big variation in how people react to tinnitus. It may surprise you to learn that most people with tinnitus get along with it without any great distress. Other people suffering from tinnitus may experience feelings of anxiety or depression. They can become withdrawn or alternatively very restless. They frequently complain of poor sleep, difficulty in everyday functioning, or a reduced quality of life. Some people feel the need for antidepressants, sleeping pills or other tranquilizers.

For example, one of our patients, Bill (a well-educated, high-earning financier) became highly anxious when he developed tinnitus. He took sick leave from work and withdrew from his family and friends and spent periods of time in bed or lying on his sofa. His physician prescribed tranquillizers and antidepressants. This may sound very familiar but remember that most people with tinnitus are emotionally fine. It's also the case that you can have a lot of problems with your tinnitus for a limited period of time and then move on to a calmer period during which you are much less annoyed by it. Given the choice, obviously most people would rather not have tinnitus; but after an initial stress reaction to it they carry on leading normal healthy and fulfilling lives and don't attend tinnitus clinics. Many people who do come to our clinics suppose that suffering is an inevitable consequence of having tinnitus. How often have we, as clinicians, heard a patient say: "Of course I feel like this. I have tinnitus! How could I feel any other way?" People see an inevitable link between having tinnitus and feeling bad, but the link is not inevitable. It is possible to have tinnitus and still be okay. Remember, most people with tinnitus are okay! After an initial stress reaction they simply stop reacting to the same old boring tinnitus sound and become largely unaware of their tinnitus for most of the time. This process is called habituation and occurs naturally so long as you regard the tinnitus as meaningless. Many people are greatly relieved to hear this. Some of our patients, like Bill, however, protest by saying: "Sure, other people might be okay, but they can't have bad tinnitus. Mine is really bad and anyone who has what I have in my ears/head is bound to suffer. Surely, no one could habituate to a noise like this."

The link, however, is not so inevitable. People with all kinds of tinnitus can be fine and people with all kinds of tinnitus can suffer. Do not despair if you have tinnitus. The outlook is very good. You too can get to a point where tinnitus does not play a prominent role in your life. Many of our patients find this hard to believe in the early stage, but it's true.

## Where does the Reaction come from?

The evidence is that psychological processes, and not just physiological ones, make a real difference to whether or not habituation takes place. Distress due to tinnitus involves a lot of worry or overly negative thinking about the symptom, a change in the way the person does things, a high level of stress arousal or tension in the person's system, and a decline in their mood. Let's look at each of these in turn.

### Thinking about Tinnitus

This is the most important bit; once this part is understood everything else falls into place. Psychologists believe that how you think about things determines how you feel. We believe that how you think about what is happening to you can be more important than what is actually happening. At first this may seem unlikely and it certainly needs careful explanation.

Different people might think about the same thing in different ways and therefore feel very differently about it. For example, a person who really believes that his or her tinnitus is a symptom of a brain tumor is likely to feel very anxious as a consequence of that thought. When his tinnitus first began, our patient Bill thought his tinnitus was the result of poisoning from a radioactive dye he received when he had an MRI scan. It's easy to understand that while he thought this and had the words "poison" and "radioactive" spinning around his mind he felt highly anxious. Fortunately, it was quite straightforward to reassure him about this. However, this is not done just by convincing the person that he is wrong.

On the contrary, a cognitive perspective calls for a collaborative stance where evidence is reviewed and all worries and concerns are taken for real until they have been carefully scrutinized. A person who thinks that tinnitus is of no significance for their health or well-being is likely to feel much calmer. It's also the case that one person might think about a thing in different ways at different times. For example, most of us have had the experience of worrying about a problem in the middle of the night. The problem can seem huge and insurmountable and we feel terrible. By lunchtime the next day the problem may not have gone away but it may seem more manageable and we feel less terrible. We can therefore think differently about the same problem at different times and it is the thinking that leads to us feeling stressed or not.

We also know that when people are stressed they think about things in an overly negative way, that is, they drop into "middle of the night" thinking most of the time—day and night. This is not to say that people are foolish to see problems where none exist, but rather we all are prone to see danger. Seeing danger can help us stay alive. The problem comes about when "middle of the night" thinking begins to take over and leads us to become overly negative about problems. Then we end up suffering more than we need to. Although Bill was easily reassured about not having been poisoned, he developed several new ideas about his tinnitus. He went to a wedding party and was seated next to a band that played very loudly. He thought that the noise would make his tinnitus worse and quickly left. Sure enough, his tinnitus was more intrusive when he left, but later it did go back to normal. He then assumed that any everyday loud sounds would make his tinnitus worse and that his tinnitus would continue to grow and grow until he became a bed-bound invalid. He told himself that he could no longer enjoy life. When he saw retired people walking in the street an image came to his mind of himself as an older person unable to function because of tinnitus. When he had this image he was overcome by feelings of anxiety and sadness.

Most people will experience some tinnitus when exposed to very loud sounds such as those produced by a band at a wedding. As long as the exposure is not too long or loud then the tinnitus will usually disappear again. Bill took his (normal) experiences with the band and generalized the idea to a very wide range of everyday settings. In a nutshell, he over-generalized the idea. This is something that can happen to any of us when under stress.

Our thoughts can become distorted in a number of ways, for example, seeing one or a few negative events as a never-ending pattern or thinking of things in all or nothing terms. Once our thoughts take on a "middle of the night" distortion, then a vicious cycle of negative thoughts and negative mood is set up. When tinnitus is involved in this, the person can have a very bad time. Some people will say that they don't know what they think about tinnitus and that they try to not think about it. It's important to remember that if you're feeling bad about your tinnitus, it's because you do have ideas about it and those ideas are worrying you. Research has told us that people who suffer with tinnitus think about it much more than people who have tinnitus but do not complain about it (Hallam et al., 1984).

The key facts are that many people have tinnitus but not everyone suffers with it. The evidence indicates that when a person does suffer, it is less to do with the psychophysical aspects of the tinnitus and more to do with the worry about it. When a person drops into overly negative or "middle of the night" thinking about tinnitus, then he or she will suffer. Now let's talk more about this suffering.

### A Decline in Mood

Worrying about tinnitus triggers a number of other processes. The most obvious one is a decline in the person's mood. For many people this takes the form of feeling anxious or nervous. Bill's original belief that he had been poisoned led him to feel anxious and angry. Later, his belief that everyday loud sounds would damage his hearing system and worsen his tinnitus led him to feel more anxious. Anyone who really believed this idea would feel anxious. Holding other beliefs will lead to other types of mood. It is common for people suffering with tinnitus to complain of feeling depressed, sad, irritated, anxious, frightened, panicky, agitated, angry, ashamed, or some other unpleasant mood. What mood you feel will depend on what you are saying to yourself about the tinnitus. Once a negative mood takes hold it has a reinforcing effect on negative thinking. When we feel depressed we're more likely to have depressive thoughts. When we feel anxious we're more likely to have anxious thoughts, and so on. How we think about things including tinnitus really does depend on "what side of the bed we got out of."

## High Level of Arousal

Negative thoughts not only lead us to feel anxious, angry or depressed, they also lead to a change in the level of stress arousal in our bodies. The physical changes in arousal are an integral part of the emotional experience. When we're in an anxious mood we also have changes in our body, such as increased heart rate, increased muscle tension (and with it a feeling of tension and sometimes pain, typically in the head, neck and shoulders), increased breathing rate, increased digestion rate (although in the upper gut things slow down and we feel butterflies or nausea) and with it an increase in the frequency and urgency with which we need the toilet.

Many of our tinnitus patients complain of such symptoms, particularly headache or pains around the ear and a general feeling of being tense. There are many other physical changes that can take place in such circumstances. For example, this increase in physical arousal can make it more difficult to sleep. These changes can be very frightening if you don't know what's going on and mistake the symptoms for illness, or you worry that they'll have some other damaging effect on you.

Our patient Bill experienced a sensation like a tight band around his head, felt incredibly tense, and suffered with nausea and diarrhea. In this way there can be a vicious cycle between negative thoughts and physical symptoms of stress arousal. Increased arousal also has other less physically obvious effects. In particular, increased arousal causes a person's attention to focus ever more narrowly on the thing that is perceived as a threat. As a result, a person who believes that tinnitus is a threat to well-being will focus attention on tinnitus to the exclusion of other things. This is known as selective attention and its effect is very unhelpful in this situation. Just imagine what would happen if you lay on your bed for fifteen minutes and did nothing but focus your attention on your tinnitus. It would surely seem much louder and be much more intrusive.

We believe that it is this process that leads people to describe their tinnitus in terms such as "like a jet engine" or "like a road drill." It also leads people to hear their tinnitus even when other loud noises are present.

## Changes in Behavior

Most people who perceive themselves to be in danger will try to do something to keep safe from that danger. This is usually very helpful, but when the perceived threat results from thinking about things in a "middle of the night" way, then actions that keep you safe are likely to be unhelpful. Remember, "middle of the night" thinking leads to problems being seen as bigger than they really are. In such circumstances, actions that keep you safe are likely to mean that you will not find out that you've overestimated the extent of the problem; that is, that you're caught up in an anxious or depressed thinking trap. In this way the overly negative thoughts will be kept alive.

For example, Bill's belief that everyday loud sounds would damage his auditory system and worsen his tinnitus led him to keep away from such noises. He avoided noise as much as possible, even to the point that he insisted that his family be as quiet as possible. His children had to play quietly in another room and his wife would wait until he was out to use the vacuum cleaner. This safety behavior meant that he didn't find out that everyday loud sounds would not damage his auditory system. Keeping safe meant that Bill's overly negative thoughts were kept alive. These thoughts went on provoking his anxious mood and the stress arousal in his body and his focus on tinnitus. Bill kept his environment quiet but it is common for people who are suffering with tinnitus to do the opposite and avoid quiet situations at all costs. This can be equally unhelpful if it prevents you finding something out or testing an idea. For example, "My tinnitus will be unbearable if I don't have background sound and I'll be unable to function."

### What Needs to Happen to Change these Reactions?

If you're distressed by tinnitus, the key to reducing that distress is changing how you think about it. There are no rules that dictate how this can be achieved but there are some tried and trusted methods. The first thing to do is find out what's going through your mind about it. This might be done through discussion with your psychologist or tinnitus therapist. It can also be done by noting what goes through your mind when you're feeling distressed by it. (There are some ideas about identifying worrying thoughts in the next section.)

You're almost certainly just accepting the thing(s) that you're saying to yourself about tinnitus as accurate or correct. Although these ideas will seem very compelling, you must remember that they are ideas rather than facts. Also remember that if you're feeling very distressed, then these ideas may be the result of "middle of the night" thinking. They need to be tested rather than just accepted. You may be able to test out how accurate they are by discussing them with your therapist. Bill was able to change his ideas about his tinnitus resulting from radioactive dye poisoning through discussion with one of us and he felt better for it. Many ideas can be tested during discussion. For example, "It's not fair that I have tinnitus" or "My tinnitus will lead me to go mad." The strength of some other ideas, such as Bill's idea that "noise will make my tinnitus worse," can be weakened by discussion but would probably not change substantially unless he changed his behavior, for example, by deliberately spending time in a noisy environment. Bill did this and his tinnitus did get more intrusive, but he realized that this happened because he was anxious and checking it; it then went back to normal after a little while. When your ideas and your behavior change, your mood will change and your level of arousal will decline. You may want to help reduce the arousal by also learning some proper relaxation exercises. When the thoughts, behavior, arousal and mood change, the tinnitus becomes less intrusive and more an innocuous part of the background.

### How can I Help Myself?

There are a number of things you can do to help yourself as you'll see. We'll present some of them here.

## Identify Your Thoughts about Tinnitus

The starting point is to find out what your ideas about tinnitus are. Ask yourself: "What is going through my mind about tinnitus?" A good time to ask this is when your tinnitus is intrusive and you're feeling distressed. It is at this time that the thoughts will be easier to "catch." It's best to try to write the thoughts down rather than trying to keep them in your mind and remember them. Writing thoughts down seems to make a real difference. Keep a pencil and paper on hand and try to write things down as soon after the event as possible. At this stage try not to write down a reasoned argument about what's happening; just try to catch the unhelpful thought. Becoming aware of the content of your thoughts can be a difficult thing and many people find that it takes practice. Typical worrying thoughts that people have about tinnitus include:

- I will end up having a nervous breakdown;
- this will affect my physical health;
- tinnitus has affected my brain and my ability to think;
- I will go deaf;
- life will never be the same again;
- I will never get any peace and quiet;
- I can't enjoy things now;
- I will never be able to enjoy life again;
- I can't do normal things anymore;
- I must avoid loud sounds;
- I must avoid silence;
- other people don't understand;
- it's not fair that this happened to me.

These are, of course, just examples of the types of thoughts about tinnitus that people have. You may not see your own worries listed here or you may hold similar ideas expressed in different words. It's important to work out what your own ideas are about tinnitus. Don't try to produce a carefully reasoned piece of prose about your tinnitus. Rather, try to discover the actual words or images that go through your mind. These words and images may be poorly articulated and fleeting, but they're the ones that cause the emotional pain that lead to the arousal and ultimately that keep you focused on your tinnitus. Generally, the thoughts of people who are suffering with tinnitus reflect despair, persecution, hopelessness, loss of enjoyment, a desire for peace and quiet, and beliefs that others do not understand (Andersson et al., 2005). Other common themes are resentment about persistence of tinnitus, a wish to escape it, and worries about health and sanity.

Sometimes people are more aware of the feeling or mood they're experiencing than of the thought that provoked it. Tuning into the emotion can give you a clue about what the thought might be.

Generally:
- an anxious mood is triggered by ideas that things are going to go wrong;
- a depressed or low mood is triggered by ideas that things already have gone wrong or something has been lost;
- anger is triggered by the idea that someone has broken the rules or done something wrong;
- guilty feelings are triggered by the idea that you did something wrong.

Another way of identifying thoughts about tinnitus is to ask yourself what are you doing, or not doing, because of your tinnitus, and then ask why you are acting like this. It's often necessary to ask yourself what the implication of your idea is. For example, if the first idea that you write down is "my tinnitus will never go away," then it's useful to ask, "What does this mean for me?" If the answer is something like, "It means I'll never be able to enjoy things anymore," then this idea is the one that you'll need to work on. It's sometimes necessary to keep asking what the implication is of each refinement of the idea in order to get to the heart of the matter. This approach to questioning ideas is called "laddering" because you're taking the idea to a new rung each time. Sometimes, ideas combine to create a mix of feelings. For example, if you believe that having tinnitus means that you've lost the ability to have peace and quiet, you're likely to feel sad, but you may also feel anxious if you then believe that a lack of peace and quiet will drive you mad.

Once the ideas have been identified, it's helpful to make the link between the ideas and the mood you feel. For example, just note that the idea, "Life will never be the same again," is triggering a depressed mood or the idea "Tinnitus will lead me to have a nervous breakdown," is triggering an anxious mood. Understanding that ideas trigger moods can help you change things. Just saying, "I feel down and I don't know why," is unlikely to help you change.

### "Middle of the Night" Thinking

It is also helpful to remember that how you feel can also influence the thoughts you have. Remember, feeling bad can lead to "middle of the night" thinking. Consider whether your ideas fit into one of these patterns. The most usual patterns of "middle of the night" thinking include:

- over-generalizing;
- All or Nothing thinking;
- ignoring positive information;
- minimizing the importance of positive information while magnifying the importance of other negative information;
- using a mental filter wherein a small piece of information is dwelt upon and colors your vision of reality like a drop of ink that discolors an entire beaker of water;
- emotional reasoning—you believe that because you feel something is true it must be true;
- jumping to conclusions by making negative interpretations without having firm evidence to support the conclusions.

Realizing that an idea fits one of the well-recognized patterns can be helpful; it can make change easier. Over-generalization and all-or-none thinking were characteristics of Bill's thinking. Understanding that his thinking was skewed in these ways encouraged him to look for alternative ways of thinking about his tinnitus. Sometimes, however, it can be difficult to decide which pattern best fits the picture and sometimes ideas don't seem to fit any of these typical patterns. At such times it may be enough to simply ask, "How is this way of thinking making me feel?"

### Looking for a More Balanced Perspective

Our approach to tinnitus is one of Cognitive Behaviorial Therapy (CBT). CBT is not simply about looking on the bright side of things, positive thinking or pretending that bad things are not happening. It's about seeing if there is any other way of looking at what's happening to you. It's about taking an accurate or balanced perspective. Because stress pushes us in to "middle of the night" thinking, we often end up having overly negative ideas about things like tinnitus. This is the same thing as inaccuracy or imbalance in thinking. CBT is not about ignoring the negative but restoring the balance so that your ideas can be more accurate. Even though it acknowledges negative information, an accurate perspective will lead you to feel better than an overly negative one.

Sometimes just becoming aware of your thoughts and articulating them is enough to see that they're overly negative and to cause them to change. Often, however, the ideas need further consideration because they seem so compelling. There are no rules about how you should further consider your ideas or achieve a balanced perspective. You can try anything you think may help you find out if your ideas are accurate, but we have listed below a few questions that many people find a useful starting point:

- What is the evidence in support of this idea?
- What is the evidence that this idea is not true?
- What is the worst thing that could happen?
- What would I say to a friend?
- What would a friend say to me?
- If I was not feeling so stressed what would I think?
- Are there any other reasons why I might feel like this?

For example, when Bill recognized that one of the ideas troubling him was that he "could not enjoy life," he set about looking at the evidence for and against this idea. First, he made a list of the evidence in support of the idea. For example, he had felt tired more often recently and he had taken to his bed on a number of occasions and found it difficult to do some things that he normally found easy. He also felt anxious when entering noisy situations. He then made a list of things that did not support the idea; for example, a list of times when he had enjoyed himself. He noted that he had enjoyed being with a friend and enjoyed gardening. He also enjoyed shopping with his wife. He managed to play with the children and this was not great but okay. Bill had to be careful of "all or nothing" thinking.

Enjoying things to some extent, but not fully, is not the same thing as not enjoying them. Thinking about such things in this careful way is important. By comparing his lists Bill was able to modify his belief that he did not enjoy things. His new idea was: "Things are not what they were but they're not all bad, I still enjoy quite a lot of things." This idea was less distressing than his original all-or-nothing thinking. Remember, write down the ideas and the evidence for and against them or the things that you would say to a friend.

Writing has a more powerful effect than just trying to hold the ideas in your mind. Many negative thoughts can be addressed in this way and you can weaken or break the hold that they have over you. The result will be less distress, less arousal and less focus on tinnitus.

## Changing your Behavior

Many ideas can be changed by the sort of careful reflections described in the previous section, but some ideas stubbornly remain in spite of careful consideration. Sometimes a person can intellectually understand that ideas are not accurate but nonetheless continue to be convinced by them at an emotional level. That is, you can know something with your head but not with your heart. Often the accuracy of a belief can be tested only by trying things out. Frequently this means doing things in a different way from our usual habit. Because our distressing ideas seem so compelling we usually behave as if those ideas are true and we act in ways that we think will keep us safe by stopping a bad thing from happening or limiting the anxiety we feel.

Unfortunately, keeping safe in this way helps to maintain the "middle of the night" thinking and therefore the distress and focus on tinnitus is fuelled. Bill was told by his audiologist that everyday loud sounds would not damage his auditory system and would not worsen his tinnitus. He accepted this intellectually but still felt anxious about noise and avoided it. He also realized that his life had become very restricted and he and his family were suffering as a result of his own idea about this. He was therefore faced with two competing ideas - his own and his audiologist's. He believed it was worth the risk of testing out the ideas in practice by going to a noisy place. If he was right and his tinnitus worsened it would be awful, but if his audiologist was right, his life would radically change for the better. He decided to go to the cinema knowing that the anxiety and focus on his tinnitus might make it temporarily a little worse.

This is exactly what happened. The slight increase in the intrusiveness of his tinnitus was short-lived. He tried a few more similar experiments with equal success. He now knew that every day sounds were harmless; he knew this with his head and his heart. The restrictions on his life lifted and his focus on tinnitus went. He still had tinnitus if he listened for it but he no longer had a problem. Bill's life radically improved and he went back to work and in due course he came off his medications. Testing out your ideas by doing things differently leads to the most powerful change. Identify what your distressing thought is about tinnitus and work out what you're doing to keep yourself safe. Then work out what you could do differently that would test this idea.

This might involve doing something differently or stopping doing something, for example, stop keeping busy all the time. Watch out for "middle of the night" thinking when devising the experiment. All or nothing thinking can lead you to suppose that extreme changes are needed to test your ideas; this is not necessarily so. Once you've decided what changes to make then make some careful predictions about what will happen. Then try things out and note exactly what does happen and consider what the outcome means for your original idea. In a nutshell, act as your own therapist.

## Changing Arousal Level and Mood

Arousal levels can be reduced directly by learning and practicing some proper relaxation exercises. The term "relaxation" is used in a special sense in this context. It's not about relaxing in an everyday sense, for example, sitting in the garden or putting your feet up with a couple of beers and watching a game. There are a number of approaches to therapeutic relaxation. We recommend learning progressive muscle relaxation. This involves gentle tensing and relaxing exercises that will change the state of affairs in your body.

These exercises are not about adopting a special mental or spiritual state but are straightforward mechanical exercises that lower the level of muscle tension. This in turn reduces the level of arousal in the whole system. There are many places where these exercises can be learned and there are many tape or CD versions available. Occasionally people do find these exercises difficult, often because of physical restrictions, and then we suggest an approach called autogenic relaxation that involves relaxing through the power of imagination. Again instructions in this can be found on tape or CD. Learning relaxation is something that many people do early on in therapy. Changing how you think about tinnitus, changing how you act and practicing relaxation will lead to changes in your mood. Gentle exercise will also improve mood.

## How can a Psychologist Help?

Many people are successful in changing their reactions to tinnitus by going through the processes outlined in this chapter. It can, however, be difficult to understand your reactions and change them on your own. Professional help can make a real difference. There are different schools of psychology and we recommend that you consult a psychologist trained in Cognitive Behavior Therapy (CBT). At the time of writing few cognitive behavior therapists specialize in treating people with tinnitus but most should be able to apply their CBT skills to the problem and help a person with tinnitus.

For help in finding a cognitive behavior therapist in your area consult the American Association for Behavioral and Cognitive Therapies (www.aabt.org) or the British Association of Behavioral and Cognitive Psychotherapists (www.babcp.com). The therapist will help you understand what is going through your mind about your tinnitus. They will ask you about your tinnitus and more particularly about your reactions to it. They will listen carefully to how you talk about it and reflect back to you the things that you are saying. In this way you can both come to understand what's going through your mind about tinnitus and your reaction to it. Having another person listening and discussing your problems can lead to a much more objective view of your situation. The therapist will help you arrive at a clear understanding of what is happening to you and how the different pieces of your jigsaw fit together. On the basis of this they'll set you homework tasks. The homework will help you find out more about your thoughts and reactions to tinnitus. The therapist will also help you to discover whether your thoughts about tinnitus are accurate.

A therapist can be enormously helpful when it comes to planning how to do things differently so that your ideas can be tested. Many people think that psychology is just common sense, but very often it's much more involved than that. Many of the processes involved are actually counter-intuitive. After all, if it was all just common sense wouldn't you have sorted out the problem yourself? A psychologist will have expert knowledge of the processes that lead to distress and of the things that make people psychologically well. Applying such knowledge to your problems with tinnitus can be invaluable.

Many people get tinnitus for the first time during or after a period of high stress. Alternatively a person's tinnitus may get much more intrusive during a period of stress. It's often the case that when these other problems are addressed the tinnitus problem reduces. The therapist can help with this. If you have thoughts of harming yourself then it's very important that you seek professional help. We all make certain assumptions about the world and our place within it (for example, it's very important to never let people down) and on the basis of these assumptions we have rules about how we run life ("I must always do my best, work hard and make everything okay.") It's often the case that a person has big problems with tinnitus because assumptions about the world are too inflexible or because it makes it difficult to live by such strict rules. These beliefs are often deep-seated and hard to recognize without professional help. A therapist will help you understand these processes and decide if your life would be better if you changed them. Recognizing and changing these patterns will not turn you into someone else but can make life a lot less stressful.

Not only can a therapist bring objectivity and expert knowledge to your situation but there's a strong therapeutic effect of having someone else listen to and understand your concerns in a warm and supportive atmosphere. The therapist will help motivate you as well as support you in your efforts to change. Consulting a psychologist does not mean that you're crazy. Psychologists work with all kinds of people and all kinds of problems (not just severe mental health problems). Nor does it mean that you've given in to your tinnitus. Rather, it's the start of a new approach to overcoming the problem of your tinnitus.

## Summary

Tinnitus is important not because it exists but because of what you believe it does to you or will do to you. These ideas are not always accurate. If you can change the ideas you will change your reaction to tinnitus and you will be less aware of it.

# References

Andersson, G., Baguley, D. M., McKenna, L., & McFerran, D. J. (2005). Tinnitus: A Multidisciplinary Approach. London: Whurr.

Hallam, R. S., Rachman, S., & Hinchcliffe, R. (1984). Psychological aspects of tinnitus. In S. Rachman (Ed.), Contributions to Medical Psychology (Vol. 3, pp. 31-53). Oxford: Pergamon Press.

# Recommended Reading

Hallam, R. S. (1989). Living with Tinnitus: Dealing with the Ringing in your Ears. Wellingborough: Thorsons.

Henry, J., & Wilson, P. (2002). Tinnitus: A Self-Management Guide for the Ringing in your Ears. Boston: Allyn & Bacon.

McKenna, P., & Andersson, G. (2003). Psychological aspects of hearing impairment and tinnitus. In L. Luxon, J. M. Furman, A. Martini & D. Stephens (Eds.), Textbook of Audiological Medicine. Clinical Aspects of Hearing and Balance (pp. 593-601). London: Martin Dunitz Publishers.

# CHAPTER SIX

# Your Life and Tinnitus

## Anne-Mette Mohr, MA

*Psychologist, Interdisciplinary Health Clinic, Copenhagen*

---

**Anne-Mette Mohr** is a Clinical Psychologist and licensed existential psychotherapist. From 1995 she was the Head of a National Counseling Service aimed at person with tinnitus and hearing loss. During that time Anne-Mette Mohr counseled tinnitus patients; developed courses and established a telephone-counseling service aimed at distressed tinnitus-patients. She also developed an education for hearing therapists treating tinnitus. Today, Anne-Mette Mohr is director of The Interdisciplinary Health Clinic doing among other things psychological treatment on tinnitus. At regular intervals Anne-Mette Mohr lectures upon psychological treatment of tinnitus both in Europe and USA. Recently she has contributed to the book, Tinnitus Treatment (RS Tyler, Ed.).

---

## The End is Where We Start

Tinnitus can be quite an overwhelming experience that may have a major impact on all aspects of your life. Since the onset of tinnitus many of my patients experience that their daily life now consists of almost nothing else but the intrusive sound(s) and their constant and hopeless fight of reducing the impact of tinnitus. If this is how you're doing it is quite natural that you, in addition, will feel anxious, worried, stressed, emotionally unstable with emotions going from anger to grief, hopelessness, meaninglessness and aloneness. Because how can one imagine existing in life with nothing else but the disturbing and invading sound of tinnitus?

Therefore, when tinnitus patients come to me for psychological treatment, they have the feeling that they have come to a dead end. They cannot see the possibility of a new start. This chapter addresses patients who feel like this, who are suffering from tinnitus.

In most of this chapter I will let my patients speak through me. In this way I want to describe how tinnitus sufferers initially experience their tinnitus and how it influences the different dimensions of their lives. Perhaps you'll recognize some elements of your own story in my description. Perhaps you'll find out that you're not alone in your experience and that your reactions are known and natural. Also I want to describe the typically needs of tinnitus patients bringing some practical (and non-psychological) suggestions on how to meet these.

In order to give you an idea on how psychological therapy can help, the last part of this chapter is devoted to describe the therapeutic course of one of my tinnitus patients, Martin. You'll follow him in his travel from the point of being fixated on tinnitus to a new point where life came to overshadow his tinnitus so much that it ceased troubling and worrying him.

Martin's therapeutic course and outcome in many ways represent that of most of my patients. Patients like Martin repeatedly have shown me that if they expand their fixated focus from tinnitus to exploring the way they presently are living their life, many unknown resources and possibilities emerge that make it possible for them to co-exist peacefully with tinnitus. This typically is one outcome of psychological therapy. Many of my patients also realize they can co-exist with tinnitus; through tinnitus they have gained an enriching perspective on their life. In other words, they have moved from a position where they - due to tinnitus - could not imagine a life really worth living, to a position where tinnitus is present and life indeed is worth living.

I hope to be able to give you an understanding of how this can happen. I will also try to provide you with hope through this chapter. To make you trust that each dead end contains the possibility for a new and fruitful beginning.

## Your Life and Tinnitus

In order to describe how tinnitus can influence your life I'll use a framework stemming from the existential approach (Deurzen, 2007). According to this framework, each human being is involved in four basic dimensions of human existence: the physical, social, private and ideological world. This framework provides the psychologist and the patient with a kind of map that, during therapy, can be used quite well to grasp all the levels on which tinnitus cause trouble to the patient's life. It can also be used to support you in developing the many opportunities that are typically present in each dimension, but hasn't come to life yet. As written earlier, this is a very important step if you are to be freed of the negative influence of tinnitus.

In the physical dimension we have access to the world through our bodies, Metaphorically speaking, our body is the vessel through which we experience the physical world. This happens through our bodies' sense organs: vision, hearing, the feeling of touch, taste, the sense of movement.

When exploring the influence of tinnitus in your physical world, what typically appears is that for a substantial part of the time you cannot hear or see beyond tinnitus. Thus the former ability to sense and enjoy the world through all senses is narrowing, because dealing with tinnitus is stealing all the attention. Where previously hearing was an expanding door to the world that made it possible to understand and appreciate what was going on out there, now with tinnitus, the door has become narrower. Some of my patients metaphorically say that it's as if tinnitus lies between them and the world like a kind of disturbing spam filter. For instance, hearing through tinnitus can make it more difficult to perceive and decode what is being said. Some sounds from the external world may temporarily enhance tinnitus. Some sounds, that before were just sounds, may now sound unpleasant. When waking up at night, the first thing heard is not the pleasant and peaceful sound of the night, but tinnitus. Its presence may even hinder the return of your necessary and restorative sleep. As a result, your body during daytime can feel exhausted and tired. Many of my patients are experiencing tinnitus as something that is threatening their existence: it deprives them from the former uncomplicated access to the physical world and from the restorative sleep (that otherwise perhaps might have given them power to surrender to the tinnitus).

The brain will interpret your experience, metaphorically speaking, as a dangerous intruder. For example, like a wild animal that has to be killed in order for you to survive. As a result, the brain will initiate release of stress hormones, putting the sense organs on red alert. Now the ability to see clearly what is approaching in front of you is enhanced. However, your normal ability to see peripherally is decreasing. The sense of hearing is turned up in order to enhance the ability to determine from which direction the "wild animal" is approaching (this will make the tinnitus seem louder). The muscles tense up in order to increase the muscular power (so that "the animal" effectively can be killed).

The tinnitus-suffering patient whose brain is reacting like this will thus experience increased tinnitus, lack of overview, muscular tension and in the longer run, muscular pain.

To sum up: the body's way of perceiving and reacting to the physical world risk changing from being unproblematic to being something worrying and stressful. Hence, tinnitus may very well have an impact on your physical being in the world.

The second basic dimension, the social world, contains all aspects of the daily life's social interaction. Tinnitus may have an influence on how you interact with people at work, with your friends and family. Because tinnitus is invisible to others, you're not sure if they understand your condition even though you might have explained it to them. This happens because you look the same as before, yet feel very different: it's not visible to others that you're terribly bothered (like it would have been had you for instance broken your leg or caught a cold).

Some patients find that the discrepancy between how they feel and how they look is difficult to handle. A draining discussion within themselves often takes place:

- Shall I be honest and tell the truth, or shall I rather just tell what I think most people want to hear (I'm fine, how are you)?
- If I tell the truth, will I be able to cover-up emotional re-
- actions like tears or sadness (which can be unpleasant and intimidating both for me and my surroundings)?
- How will people look at me if I show emotional reactions?
- Will they look at me as someone weak or hysterical?
- Will they avoid me?
- How will it be next time we meet?

Some of my patients doubt whether their friends and family will believe them in how they actually feel, while others speculate whether the friends and family will think that they want to be "interesting" and attract attention.

Tinnitus may be so disturbing and anxiety-provoking that you worry about whether you'll be able do your work, and when you're not working you may feel so worried and exhausted that you neither can find the energy to contribute to anything nor enjoy pleasant interactions with others. You may start regarding yourself as someone who others perceive as some kind of challenge to be with.

Your relation to, and view about your healthcare professionals, like for instance your audiologist or otologist, might also change through your tinnitus. Your hope might have been that your health-care professional could cure tinnitus, or at least do something to you to reduce the suffering. Now you may realize that sometimes, the professional stand is in the same line as you, not knowing what to do. You may feel dismissed through the well-known statement: "You've got to learn to live with it." Perhaps what you need is at least some understanding of what you're going through (which would make you feel less alone).

These are some examples of how tinnitus may have an influence on your social world, making your relationship to yourself and others much more complicated than they used to be.

Our private world is yet another dimension of human existence in which tinnitus may have huge impact. Our private world is where we experience closeness to ourselves and to other important individuals (like our family). Included in the dimension of our private world are our ideas, thoughts, feelings, hopes, our basic identity and even intimacy with ourselves.

Before getting tinnitus, you were able to enjoy your free hours alone or enjoy the closeness to your spouse or children. Now, your leisure time may be increasingly filled with activities that are intended to somehow distract you from tinnitus, to get rid of it or finding a way to learn to live with it. As a consequence, you may find yourself spending hours on the Internet trying to find the cure, hope, as well as the experience and knowledge shared by co-sufferers. Your identity may change from one of being healthy and well-functioning to one of feeling ill or handicapped. You may feel less worthy, insecure, alone—like an alien. You may experience difficulties being "your good old self." Before, you were able to nurture you spouse and kids giving them all the best of you, while now, you may feel a burden to them because you cannot help asking for certain consideration due to your tinnitus (for example, needing more quietness, less socializing, fewer mutual activities). Your inability to participate as much in the life of your family as well as your inability to give them your closeness as much as you would like to may make you feel like a failure. You may start speculating on how much more your family can put up with. You may feel both depressed and sad.

These are some examples of how my patients experience tinnitus in their private world. The fourth dimension, the ideological world, is where our values, ideas and beliefs about life belong. Here we create meaning for ourselves and make sense of things. Religious beliefs, spirituality, a feeling of being connected to something bigger that is beyond our control also fall under this dimension. Many of my tinnitus patients tell me how much influence their condition has on their ideas about how life should be. Like most of us, they've had thoughts about how life should unfold itself, what makes life meaningful and worth living, where they want to go, what they want to achieve sometime in the future. They've had a general feeling of control - that they were able to keep the dangers and threats at a safe distance. With tinnitus in the picture, some of these patients feel that their possibilities of carrying out their ideas and visions grow narrower or are disappearing. Life seems increasingly meaningless.

Rhetorical questions like "why me" can reflect your need to find some kind of meaning with what is happing to you. If meaning could be found, perhaps the situation would be easier to accept. Some patients grieve over the loss of silence, over the new and more troublesome way of hearing or even over the loss of the "good old self" that they used to be. Some patients feel that the old well-known jigsaw puzzle that once constituted a coherent life simply has broken into pieces.

Actually these reactions together constitute an existential crisis that needs to be resolved. If the crisis is worked through carefully, the patient can be imparted with possibilities of personal and interpersonal development. If the crisis however is ignored or not understood, and thus not adequately acted upon, this may result in a temporary fixation on a seemingly "incurable" condition. This again may result in development of depression. I write "temporary" because it is my experience that when the existential issues of the crisis are addressed with the patient coming to terms with them, the fixation disappears and the depression eases. Thus, the influence of tinnitus in the ideological world can be very powerful and shaking, initiating a crisis.

As written previously, to most patients, tinnitus does not cause much turbulence in their life. In order for you who experience no bigger problems with tinnitus, not to become worried or scared, this is very important to keep in mind when reading this chapter. However, as just described, some people experience that tinnitus has quite an impact on the four basic dimensions of their human existence. We all have to respect the individual reaction and avoid denouncing the person for whom tinnitus is difficult. Rather, help and support should be offered in order to explore whether your needs have been met and whether you need assistance in looking for possibilities that will make it possible for you to co-exist peacefully with tinnitus.

I'll now use the basic dimensions of human existence to describe which needs you may have. Also, I'll give you some examples on what typically helps the tinnitus patient.

## Your Needs as a Tinnitus Patient

### Your Needs in the Physical World

I can't remember having seen any tinnitus patient who hasn't had the need of getting a more thorough understanding of the "physiology" of tinnitus. These questions include:

- What is tinnitus?
- From where in my head is the sound generating?
- Why did I get tinnitus?
- What is the prognosis?
- Will it disappear?
- Will it get worse?
- Can I continue doing what I used to do (hobbies, work, family, etc)?
- Will it drive me crazy?"

All these questions need good and thorough explanations. Don't feel bad about having the need to want to know. It's a normal human need to see and understand the mechanism behind what is happening to us. The more we understand, the more we may be able to do something about it. If, for instance, your car has the irritating habit of stopping in the middle of crossroads, it probably won't be a good enough solution for you just to think: "What a nuisance that my car always stops in the middle of the crossroads." You'll need to know what causes the problem so you have the best possibility for doing something about it.

Thus, many tinnitus patients, as their first step, will consult an audiologist or otologist in order to find out whether the sound actually is tinnitus, to be examined in order to rule out dangerous conditions and to gain a basic understanding. However, providing the basic understanding of tinnitus as well as answering important questions are quite time-consuming. As a consequence many busy clinicians choose to make the needed examinations, only to end up saying something like, "There's no need to worry, you have to learn to live with it." Often they forget referring the patient to professionals that can provide correct information, support and knowledge on how to live with it.

If this happened to you, you'll probably have searched the Internet in order to get what the clinician didn't give you: causes, prognosis, advices, as well as positive stories, information about promising cures, and so forth. However, what you may have found has, at best, had no positive effect at all, and at worst, it may have, due to all the misinformation and horror stories, had a frightening effect. You may also have started your search for help on the Internet without initially consulting a clinician. Or you may have heard terrible things about tinnitus through friends, colleagues, magazines or television. Whatever the prehistory of your time with tinnitus, the effect of the misinformation will most likely be the same: you'll be on red alert (which will stress your body, making your muscles tense and your tinnitus sound louder).

Thus, what you're in need of is finding a professional who has time enough to offer you thorough and correct information and who can function as a guide on where to get your other possible needs met. All the misinformation, as well as all your anxious assumptions, has to be clarified and then demystified; all your questions and worries need to be dealt with. You may also need to be asked questions that can help you identify and demystify all those fears that you may carry in the back of your head without realizing it. When being alert, we human beings have a tendency to read between the lines. For example, we hear more than actually is said or meant, we make inferences that might be wrong, or we fixate on some kind of worrying expression.

Thus, if the professional says something that makes you worried, don't hesitate to get things explained once more and in another way. Some tinnitus patients find great help in bringing a friend or a relative to the session with the professional, so that this person can help support and clarify during the session as well as remember to explain later on what was said in the session.

Even if you get a thorough understanding of the physiology of tinnitus and thus realize there's no need to worry, your "intellectual" understanding may not be sufficient to make you able to push tinnitus into the background. This can be very worrying, making your body respond with the continuous release of stress hormones. And your tinnitus will as a result still be experienced as loud. One of the most helpful and preferred "tools" of my patients is *progressive muscular relaxation exercises.* This technique makes the degree of alertness (as well as the intrusiveness of tinnitus) diminish quite effectively, since it is impossible to be alert and relaxed at the same time. Learning the skills of relaxation techniques in the beginning is often a matter of "will." Your body and mind may be so alert that you have to fight to keep your concentration on the training. You'll realize how tense you are and that a state of relaxation is not just something that you easily enter. You may need to find a relaxation therapist who can teach you the techniques and support you in becoming skilled. Still you'll probably end up by realizing that this tool is both the most efficient as well as the cheapest of all tools that you've tried.

### Your Needs in the Social World

The most frequent need is to meet other patients that have found their way to coexist with tinnitus and who know what it takes to succeed. Such ex-patients can be reassuring examples, especially if they know how to confirm the difficulties it can take to succeed without scaring you, and how to offer you ideas, advice and hope. Such meetings can indeed provide you with a turning point. A side benefit is that you'll decrease your feeling of being alone since you are again a member of a group. Also your feeling of being a burden to your family and friends will diminish since your needs of talking about your situation now has been met in a qualified way.

Some patients will need to talk about their situation in their social surroundings, while others prefer abstaining from this for fear of getting stuck in the present situation or fear of getting scary stories that might negatively influence them. Quite a few people fear that talking about their situation and the worries connected to it will result in them not being able to control their emotions. They speculate whether this will make them feel humiliated or looked at it in a way that they don't want to. It's my experience that exactly these considerations can give rise to new ways of "being" which in the long-run may turn out to be quite healing. Such considerations can often be favorably discussed during therapy.

## Your Needs in the Private World

You may experience different (and perhaps even for you) quite unknown reactions toward tinnitus. You may need to find out that your reactions toward tinnitus are quite understandable and normal. Actually, it can make your situation feel worse if you are both bothered by tinnitus as well as feeling wrong about your reactions. Emotional reactions, also the dark and sad ones, are a part of the human emotional palette. There's nothing wrong with these feelings as long as you know their reason for being present. Very often my patients want these feeling to go away which normally has the opposite effect—they aggravate. Just like tinnitus itself, the more you want it to go away the more power it seems to get. In my experience, what brings movement and a resulting change to the sad feelings is when my patient and I take our time to talk these feelings through. However, if you feel that everything is grey and nothing whatsoever can make you see a glimpse of light, this might be a sign that you're at risk of developing depression. When depression disappears, the impact of tinnitus lessens. If you believe you might be depressed, consult a professional who can help you sort this out.

Some of my patients have the feeling that they're not good enough and/or clever enough, since they haven't yet been able to tame tinnitus just a little bit. If this is the situation with you, let this reproach pass you by. Changes and improvement take time and it is individual how much time you need. The amount of time is not a measure on how good or clever you are, but a measure showing how heavy the challenge of tinnitus is to you. When you have come to terms with tinnitus you can take pride in yourself that you actually were able to carry so much and yet succeeded.

## Your Needs in the Ideological World

Most of us tend to live as if nothing bad could happen to us. We may realize that bad things happen, but it's as if it happens to others. We may have an expectation that only certain unpleasant things can happen, thus being very shocked when something unpleasant like tinnitus strikes us. If this is truly how your expectations to life have been, then of course with tinnitus in the picture you can feel cheated, angry, sad or resentful. These reactions need to be taken seriously because then the issue is not only about tinnitus, but also about your whole idea of how your existence was going to unfold itself through life. Perhaps the onset of tinnitus has made you realize quite vividly the fragility of human existence, how vulnerable we are. It can give rise to anxiety to realize that even if we take great care, we cannot ultimately control what is going to happen to us or to others. The anxiety may provoke tinnitus to be experienced as more intrusive.

Thus, tinnitus can be understood not only as something happening in your ears; it also can be understood as a shaking reminder of our human existential conditions. Religious leaders, existentially oriented philosophers or psychologists constitute professionals who can support you working through existentially similar themes.

## On the Track of Finding Your Way of Coexisting with Tinnitus

You're probably already aware that there's no single model or single method that provides "the one and only" answer on how to coexist peacefully with tinnitus. Nobody has up until now provided one unequivocal answer on how everybody suffering from tinnitus can come to terms with it. However, there exist many models, methods and suggestions used by different and knowledgeable professionals. Some methods help some. Other methods help others. It's difficult to foretell which will be a better model or method for you.

As a result, you'll probably need to try different methods before you find your method of coexisting with tinnitus. And you risk trying strategies that do not meet your needs. This shall not make you stop searching, falling into pitfalls of hopelessness and helplessness. There is a method somewhere and having found your method, your way, you'll probably, like my patients, experience that the best methods are the ones that you can employ yourself and that in the long-run makes you independent of professionals like hearing therapists, physiotherapists, psychologists and so forth, as well as independent of technical devices (except for hearing aids if you have a hearing loss). I think this is a great perspective and I hope you'll keep it in mind.

During the process of coming to terms with tinnitus, you may need a guide who can provide you with hope, when hopes seem lost; reassure you when feeling down, lightening you up when darkness overshadows your ability to find possibilities. A psychologist might constitute such a guide.

Martin chose to seek psychological help. His therapeutic course is reflective of the course that most patients go through when coming to me due to troublesome tinnitus. As you'll see, the therapeutic process expanded Martin, from only having the focus on tinnitus, to how he could increase his repertoire of being in the four dimensions. Frankly, I cannot remember having had one tinnitus-suffering patient in therapy who didn't experience the same process as Martin. This is the "risk" I guess you run when consulting a psychologist – to land somewhere quite differently from where you expected. Whether this is for the good or bad is for you to judge.

### Tinnitus and the Patient's Other Story

After a rock concert five years ago, Martin got tinnitus but learned to live with it without too much trouble. However, days after his 52nd birthday he became aware of a new intrusive tinnitus sound. This he didn't understand since after the onset of tinnitus he had been very careful to protect his hearing. His audiologist couldn't establish the reason for the new sound, but very counterproductively told Martin about his own futile fight with coming to terms with it. Since tinnitus continued being very intrusive he felt increasingly worried and depressed. When finally seeking psychological help at my clinic he had started on antidepressants and also using sedatives before going to bed.

Initially in therapy Martin needed solid answers to all his questions, some mentioned earlier in this chapter. However, his intellectual understanding of the physiological side of tinnitus didn't result in a less intrusive tinnitus. Martin metaphorically expressed it as: "I can see the plate and the food but I lack the knife and fork." Thus, I suggested to Martin that we start out on an exploration of the four dimensions of his existence in order to see whether there were some hidden possibilities, when brought into light, could provide him with the "knife and fork."

Going through his way of existing in the physical world, it appeared that Martin never had given his body a chance to recover. He was devoted to his job as headmaster in an upper secondary school. He took pride in being there for the pupils and their parents, supporting them through difficult times. He also gave his leadership a high priority. He was very attentive to his teachers' needs for good leadership that could direct them through all the constant and challenging changes that the educational system continuously imposed on Danish schoolteachers. In order to act promptly on any application, his phone and mail was always open. His cell phone was very important to him and followed him everywhere. He liked to be the last man on his job and the first one to arrive. Privately he was dedicated to art executed in the third world and was chairman of a third world art association. This also demanded much time and energy. The weekends and holidays were used to fulfill the needs of his teenage son, his five-year old, a daughter and wife as well as catching up with unfinished business related to work. In order to manage everything, he went to bed very late and got up very early. He loved what he was doing and had the idea that as long as he just loved what he was doing - whatever the degree - things were okay. When he came to me, he felt angry about the impact of tinnitus that apparently blocked his ability to continue his way of existing in life

Going back in the history of his physical world, it turned out that in the last five years he had episodes of palpitations, headaches, back pain, as well as trouble with his digestion. His response to this had been one of ignorance, using medicine and linseed oil. But his approach was always full speed forward. He had never had the idea that maybe his body was signalling something to him like: "Please give me some rest," thus giving himself the possibility of responding appropriately to his body's needs.

During the psychological sessions something strange and unexpected happened to him. Tinnitus decreased and sometimes was even difficult for him to hear. Wondering about how this could be, Martin realized that when with me the focus was primarily on him and his needs, instead of finding solutions to the problems of others. This provided him with a good and calming feeling that he identified as "the core of himself." He also discovered that he allowed his body to be seated more comfortably than he normally did. For instance, he was leaning back in my settee instead of sitting on its edge. He then noticed that his breathing was more relaxed.

To see if he could develop this idea, Martin consulted my colleague, a relaxation therapist, who subsequently taught him body awareness as well as progressive muscular relaxation techniques. Between the sessions with me and her, through practicing relaxation techniques, he trained himself to place his focus on a different part of his body instead of being preoccupied with tinnitus, as well as taking focus off his different obligations connected with work, his hobbies or family. He discovered that when being intensely absorbed on doing the training, he couldn't be intensely absorbed on his tinnitus.

Ultimately, he became increasingly aware of his body's need to have some limits for his level of activity, since muscular pain, headaches as well as tinnitus decreased through the training but increased when he exceeded his physical limits.

The relaxation therapist also instructed Martin to enjoy himself in a park and listen to the different birds. He was instructed to listen carefully to each bird's song keeping account on how many different birds were singing. From time to time he shifted his focus to other pleasant sounds and then he shifted between focusing on those and on the birds' songs (exercise developed by Gerhard Hesse, Ute Pöllmann, Christina Wöhrmann, Tinnitus Klinik, Bad Arolsen, from Germany). Because the active listening to a chosen sound overshadows tinnitus, Martin learned that it was possible to listen to sounds without being bothered by tinnitus. Furthermore, by using his hearing through his "will" to listen actively, he also expanded his quality of life. Until the onset of tinnitus, most of the time he had been in contact with the world through his mind and activities, thus mainly existing only in the social world. Now, through the active involvement of his hearing, he had expanded his territory of the physical world, that up until then had been almost nonexistent. Quite paradoxically, the narrowing experience of tinnitus thus developed into a new door behind which the pleasures of listening to all the different sounds were discovered.

Tinnitus struck Martin in the heart of his social world. When coming to me, he was on sick-leave and found it almost impossible to socialize with anybody except his wife. He mainly stayed at home, fearing he might meet somebody who would doubt if he was actually doing as badly as he claimed. "I look my old self," he said to me, "so people may think I'm making all this up, but on the other hand, I don't feel up to explaining how I am." He continued by reflecting on how he normally would be the one that would help others coming to terms with their problems. It was a totally new situation for him to be the one who had problems and was in need of some kind of help. However, he simply didn't know how to let oneself be helped by others. How does one receive help? Therefore, after the onset of tinnitus he had initially carried on as he used to, being available for others. But since tinnitus hindered him like a squeaky brake, he finally went on sick leave. Thus, he went from one position, the very active one, to another position, the very passive one. A new balance on how to be in the social world obviously needed to be found.

Martin always felt called upon to be of service to others while not taking care of himself. It turned out that he had been raised by parents who both were devoted religious people, doing lots of charity work. His parents were very hardworking and humble people with the ingrained idea that they could always do better. As a result, they encouraged their four children also to do better, not praising them for what they actually did. Martin had, for instance, never in his childhood heard his parent's say, "Well done. Good boy! Now, this is as far as we can go. Let's take a well-earned break."

In other words, the parents had not taught their children when enough was enough (limitations). They had not "fed" the children with feelings of being "good enough." This was not to say that the parents hadn't done their best. This was probably exactly what they had tried to do. Martin himself said that the atmosphere in his childhood basically had been very loving. His upbringing, however, had given him the idea that you only have a right to exist through what you do and give, and not through who you are. It had provided him with a feeling of basically not being good enough (low self-esteem) as well as an uncertainty of when "good enough" was enough. This uncertainty was the generator of his constantly exceeding his limits. As a young man with lots of energy he was able to work very hard. As he got older, he required more "down time" to recover from this output of energy. In a sense, he was writing checks without putting money in the bank. As a consequence, he was depleting his mental and physical capacities. As previously described, he had for some years received signals from his body. Not responding to them might have resulted in him hearing tinnitus to which he was desperate to stop!

Examining the jigsaw puzzle of his life we found that the bits and pieces representing his desire to give and yet received little in return, along with his low self-esteem, followed him in all aspects of his social world. We also saw how his style of living made him very powerful by being a provider and feeling purposeful. On the other hand, this style of living was possibly what contributed to tinnitus.

Through therapy, new possibilities of living were explored and tried. For him to realize that his wife truly loved and appreciated him even if he was unable to function came to him as a positive surprise. Finding out that his wife for a long time had longed for a husband who would just be together with her doing nothing brought them closer.

With respect to his work, new ways of living were also explored. Here we have to remember that society today basically has the same attitude as Martin's parents had for themselves and to their children: you are what you are through how you perform. Martin realized that it would be unrealistic to undertake too many changes at one and same time. For instance, he could not just suddenly change his general way of being who he was as the head in the school without causing too much turbulence; thus he initially started out with minor changes that, for him, were quite important, such as introducing office hours where you could reach him on the telephone as well as making clear how quickly one could expect a response from him by email. In other words, he began playing with his limits. Actually, his staff reacted positively.

Martin realized that personal development always will imply interpersonal development. This made rise for new considerations about how to be a spouse, parent and boss, whether it perhaps could be fruitful to involve others and make use of their potentials instead of doing everything yourself. Martin began feeling more energetic as well as curious on how things would develop and finally went back to work. He quit the medication and found that by creating a better balance in his social world, he was able to help himself manage tinnitus. Through tinnitus, his repertoire of how to exist in the social world started and continued expanding.

In his private world, his sense of self - his identity - was explored. Martin's sense of self for his whole life had been closely connected to what he did for others, and as alluded to earlier society generally supports the kind of changes Martin sought. Of course, early on, Martin found it very difficult and challenging to create other ways of functioning.

Furthermore, when exploring his way of functioning more deeply, we found that it actually provided him with ability to covering up his feeling of not being good enough. In other words, he had the idea that as long as he was keeping busy, others wouldn't be able to see him behind his facade. When asking him what would be found had you been able to access his hidden self, he promptly compared himself to the Emperor in the fairy tale, "The Emperor's New Suit" written by the Danish writer Hans C. Andersen:

> "I basically have the feeling of wearing nothing - that I
> am nobody special - and I fear the day when everybody
> and not just the little boy will find out, when it becomes
> disclosed how little I know and how incompetent I am.
> I fear the laughter and the rejection."

If this truly was how he felt about himself you can very well understand why he chose to live the way he did. However, Martin had not realized these motives until having time as well as the need to explore the roots of his self. When he started putting words on the different bits and pieces of his life's jigsaw puzzle, his way of being in life became increasingly clear to him. Alas, in order for him to undertake some changes, it presupposed, as for most of us, a thorough knowledge of his "state of affairs." (If we don't know how things are as well as what there is, we cannot provide changes because we're in the dark.) It also presupposed an idea about how he wanted his life to be, where he - metaphorically speaking - wanted to go. He also needed go through his values in order to see whether some adjustments or changes were needed. This took him on an exploration into his ideological world.

During therapy, themes that belong to the ideological world were discussed, like human vulnerability and what's important to us in life. Here I'll just let the focus remain on one of Martin's ambiguous and important values. He wanted to be a person who "made a difference." He had outlived that value, as we've seen, through being on the spot for others. With the onset of tinnitus it became impossible for him to outlive that value the way he used to. We have to understand and respect that for many reasons it was important for Martin to experience his value in life. And even though Martin now had a deeper understanding about some psychological aspects associated with this value (for example, low self-esteem), it still remained a value that he actively decided should exist. What he needed was to find out how to express his value in new ways. Incidentally he found another way.

At a tinnitus meeting in my clinic, Martin engaged in a conversation with some patients that recently had developed bothersome tinnitus. Martin both listened to them and talked about his own experience in a very hopeful way. Later he told me that one of these persons when saying goodbye to him had expressed how much it meant to him hearing Martin's reassuring story. Martin hadn't given advice or solutions; he had just been there with them sharing their situation and this apparently had made the difference. This success gave rise for new experiments on how to make a difference.

When having recreated and expanded the ideological world, Martin ended up by finding himself in the paradoxical situation where he on the one hand would have preferred not to get tinnitus. On the other hand he would not have been without the development that took place through tinnitus. Martin realized that his personal development occurred piggybacked onto crises; that is, if we are prepared to live through risk, we might end up somewhere quite different in life. As for tinnitus, it still was heard but Martin hadn't much time to attend to it. In this way, tinnitus developed into becoming an unimportant sound with which he could peacefully coexist.

## Conclusion

I hope by now to have shown you quite clearly what my patients have shown me—how tinnitus may influence the different dimensions of their life and what the typical needs of the tinnitus patients are. I also hope to have made it clear that for some patients there's a need to create a better balance in the dimensions in order for them to be able to co-exist peacefully with tinnitus. Therefore, you have to take the whole person's being as well as his or her relation to oneself and others into consideration, not only ears and tinnitus.

## Reference

Emmy van Deurzen (2007). Existential Counselling & Psychotherapy in Practice. London: Sage Publications.

CHAPTER SEVEN

# Hearing Loss and Communication

## Christina T. Stocking, AuD
*University at Buffalo*

---

**Dr. Stocking** is a Clinical Assistant Professor at the University at Buffalo. She has been practicing audiology in a variety of clinical and educational settings since 1980. She earned her Doctor of Audiology from The Pennsylvania College of Optometry's School of Audiology in 2003, where she was awarded the Dean's Award for Academic Excellence. Dr. Stocking was instrumental in the development of a tinnitus management program at the University, where she continues to see tinnitus patients on a daily basis and conducts research in the area of tinnitus evaluation and treatment. She teaches courses and lectures on the topics of hearing loss, hearing aids, and tinnitus. Dr. Stocking would like to thank her husband and four wonderful children for their constant love and support of her work.

---

Tinnitus is an auditory phenomenon. In order to begin to understand tinnitus, you must understand how the auditory system works. My job is to teach you enough about the human auditory system to assist in this process. Chronic tinnitus almost always occurs with some sort of dysfunction of the auditory system, so we'll explore the various types and causes of hearing loss. Our sense of hearing connects us to the world and is especially important for communication, socializing and learning. Even a mild form of hearing loss can have a significant impact on communication and lifestyle, and so we'll discuss the various effects of hearing loss on daily life. And finally, because this book is about tinnitus, we'll consider the relationship between hearing loss and tinnitus.

### Why and How We Hear

Let's start with the "why." The sense of hearing, like all of our senses, is something we take for granted. Rarely do we stop to think about what it would be like not to hear. However, when we lose some of our hearing, it becomes painfully clear what an important life sustaining function it is. Many have heard the story of how Helen Keller felt about being both blind and deaf. The following is an excerpt from a personal record written by Helen Keller in 1910:

> "The problems of deafness are deeper and more complex, if not more important, than those of blindness. Deafness is a much worse misfortune. For it means the loss of the most vital stimulus—the sound of the voice that brings language, sets thoughts astir and keeps us in the intellectual company of man."
>
> (Love, 1933)

Helen Keller's sentiments speak to the higher order of hearing function, that of learning, language and social connection. However, hearing first serves a much more basic function—that of survival. Our sense of hearing at a subconscious level, serves to alert us to our environment, keeping us constantly aware of our surroundings, especially to changes in our surroundings. Without the need for conscious thought, we turn our heads toward a new sound. We know the direction from which a sound originates. Our auditory system alerts us to new and potentially dangerous sounds, while allowing us to ignore familiar or neutral sounds.

Consider early man living in the woods. Basic survival depended on his ability to be constantly aware of approaching danger, like a predator animal (or possibly a cranky neighbor into whose territory he accidentally stumbled). The snap of a twig would elicit an immediate head turn in the direction of the sound, and send signals through the man's body to be ready to fight or flee. His heart rate and breathing would quicken; blood would rush to his extremities; his other senses (vision and smell) would be heightened. All of this because an unexpected sound picked up by the human ear was enhanced by the "subconscious" part of the auditory system. Now, the signal reaches the conscious part of the auditory system - the brain - and the man recognizes the sound as that of an animal running. At about the same moment, the man turns to see that his favorite dog has followed him into the woods. He takes a deep breath, relaxes, and yells at his dog for sneaking up on him like that. As they carry on through the woods, the sound of the dog's running feet drifts back into the man's subconscious, no longer considered important to pay attention to.

The same scenario could happen to you, modern man (or woman). Picture yourself walking down a dark street in an unfamiliar neighborhood. As you pass by an alleyway, there's a sudden scuffling noise. Your auditory system prepares you just as it did the caveman, but this time you also grab on tight to your wallet or purse as you get ready to run (a more recent adaptation for survival). Happily, it's just a stray dog so you can relax.

So I think you get my point. Our hearing is essential to our survival. However, in modern times, the higher order functions of hearing are more obviously beneficial to our way of life. As infants, we begin to develop language by hearing the same speech sounds over and over. We eventually learn the patterns of speech that lead to the meaning of words. Throughout our lives, we continue to use sound to learn and understand our world. Hearing connects us to our environment and to other people. It's our primary means of social connection. If we lose even a small amount of hearing, it can have an effect on our social interactions and our sense of well-being. The additional effort required to carry on a conversation with impaired hearing can be quite stressful. Tinnitus is often an early sign of hearing loss.

If you begin to notice even a little hearing loss or tinnitus, you should have a hearing evaluation. The evaluation will be performed by an audiologist who will be able to explain the type and degree of hearing loss you have, and whether or not you're a candidate for hearing aids or other types of hearing assistance. A medical ear specialist (an *otologist* or *otolaryngologist*) will address any underlying medical conditions associated with the hearing loss. In order to understand the results of your evaluation, it would be helpful to know how the ear and auditory system works. So let's go on now to appreciate how we hear.

The first thing to understand about how we hear is that we actually "hear" with our brain. The ear that is visible on the outside of our head is just there to collect sound and direct it toward the eardrum and beyond where the process of transforming the sound into a signal that can be recognized by the brain begins. It's helpful to think about the auditory system in two main parts: the *conductive* part and the *sensorineural* part.

The conductive part of the auditory system can be thought of as the mechanical part of the ear. It includes the outer and middle ear sections. The outer ear consists of the *pinna* and the external ear canal. This is the extent of the auditory system visible to the eye.

This is represented in Figure 7-1. You'll also see the middle ear consists of the eardrum (known as the *tympanic membrane*) and an air-filled space behind the eardrum, occupied by a chain of three small bones (the *ossicles*). These three bones are named the *malleus,* the *incus,* and the *stapes.* You may have learned them as the hammer, anvil and stirrup as a child in school. The middle ear structures are collectively responsible for conducting sounds from the environment through to our inner ear where the sensory organ of hearing lies.

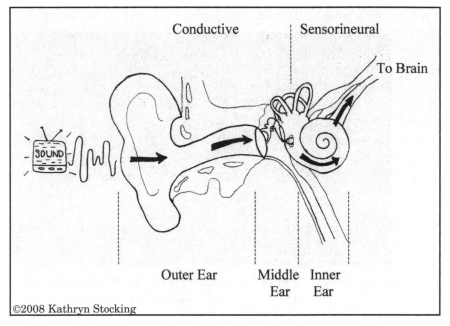

Figure 7-1: Illustration of the three basic parts of the ear

So, if we imagine a sound in the form of a wave traveling through the air, we can follow it through the conductive part of our auditory system. The sound wave is collected by the pinna, and directed into the ear canal. When it reaches the end of the ear canal, it strikes the eardrum and sets it into vibration. The sound wave has now been transformed into mechanical energy. That energy or vibration is passed along from the malleus to the incus and finally to the stapes bone which delivers the energy to the inner ear.

This brings us to the sensorineural part of the auditory system. Here, the signal will go through another transformation, from mechanical to neural energy. The sensorineural part of the ear includes 1) the *cochlea,* a snail shaped bony capsule containing the organ of hearing; 2) the *auditory nerve;* 3) the *neural pathways* traveling through the *brainstem;* and 4) the *auditory cortex* in the brain itself. The stapes bone communicates with the cochlea at a place called the *oval window.* This is a membrane that allows transfer of energy into the otherwise bony capsule of the cochlea. The cochlea is filled with fluid and contains the *organ of Corti,* which is our organ of hearing. The organ of Corti is an extremely complex structure which is still being studied by hearing scientists. A complete understanding of how this organ works is beyond the scope of this chapter. However, it's important to know that this organ contains thousands of tiny sensory *hair cells* which respond to movement and generate neural signals which are then sent via the auditory nerve and brainstem pathways up to the brain.

As we follow that sound wave, the vibrations that have traveled through the middle ear are passed into the cochlea at the oval window. Since the cochlea is filled with fluid, the vibrations form a wave action in the cochlear fluids and structures. This wave action causes the hair cells to bend. The bending of the hair cells then creates nerve impulses that are passed along to the auditory nerve, through the brainstem, and on to the brain where the nerve impulses are interpreted as sound.

Our auditory system is exquisitely designed to preserve the characteristics of sound. A sound can be described by such characteristics as pitch, loudness and timing. In the conductive part of our ear, the pattern of the sound wave is passed along and preserved as mechanical energy. Once it reaches the cochlea, this pattern must be translated into a signal the brain can process. That job begins with the hair cells. Sounds of high, middle and low pitch (frequency) stimulate hair cells at different locations in the cochlea. High frequency sounds stimulate hair cells nearer to the entrance of the cochlea while low frequency sounds affect hair cells located near the innermost end of the cochlea. Since each one of the hair cells connects to different fibers of the auditory nerve, the frequency or pitch of the sound will be passed on in a code the brain can interpret. Loudness of sound is determined by the number of hair cells stimulated and the number of impulses sent to the brain. A louder sound will cause a greater disturbance in the cochlea, thereby stimulating a greater number of hair cells and sending a larger signal to the brain. The timing of sound is also coded in the cochlea by the timing of the firing of the hair cells. Therefore, you may want to think of the organ of Corti as a translator between the physical sound and the brain.

Beyond the cochlea, the translated signal in the form of neural impulses continues along its journey to the brain through numerous nerve pathways and relay stations. Along the way, the signal is evaluated and can be enhanced or ignored before ever reaching the conscious part of the brain. (Remember the automatic reaction of early man.) Information coming from the right and left ears is shared and analyzed to determine directionality and to help extract important signals from background noise. Neural impulses that reach the brain present patterns that the brain can recognize and process as meaningful sound.

## Prevalence of Hearing Loss

Loss of function at any point along this complex auditory pathway, (from the outer and middle ear through the inner ear, through the neural pathways or at the level of brain) can disrupt the process and cause problems in our ability to interpret sound. In this section we'll look at what can go wrong within the auditory system. The more common types of hearing problems will be highlighted.

According to a survey published in 2005 (Kochkin), more than 31 million Americans have hearing loss. Here are some other interesting statistics from the National Institute on Deafness and Other Communication Disorders (http://www.nidcd.nih.gov/health/):

- about 2 to 3 out of every 1000 children in the US are born deaf or hard-of-hearing;
- hearing loss increases with age: 1.7% of children under age 18 years have hearing loss, as compared to 31% of people over the age of 65 years, and 40-50% of those over age 75 years;
- hearing loss is greater in men;
- ten million Americans have suffered irreversible noise-induced hearing loss, and 30 million more are exposed to dangerous levels each day;
- only 1 out of 5 people who could benefit from hearing aids actually wears them;
- approximately 4,000 new cases of sudden hearing loss occur each year in the US; in 9 out of 10 people experienc-

ing sudden hearing loss, the loss occurs in only 1 ear; only 10-15% of patients with sudden hearing loss know the cause;

- at least 12 million Americans have tinnitus; more than 1 million of these individuals admit that the tinnitus interferes with their lives each day.

## Types of Hearing Loss

When looking at disorders of hearing, it's helpful to divide them into categories according to what part of the ear is involved. In very general terms, hearing losses are divided into conductive and sensorineural.

### Conductive Hearing Loss

Based on what you've already learned, you know that a *conductive hearing loss* has to do with a problem involving the mechanical part of the ear; something is preventing the sound from being properly conducted through the outer or middle ear. Anything that causes blockage or adds stiffness to the conductive mechanisms can cause loss of hearing. The following descriptions are the most common causes of conductive hearing loss.

### Cerumen

In the ear canal we can sometimes accumulate enough earwax (*cerumen*) to effectively block sound from reaching the eardrum. Cerumen is our ear's way of cleaning itself. Dirt and foreign bodies are collected in the wax and gradually moved out of the ear canal through a natural migrating of the skin of the ear canal. However, occasionally this process doesn't work properly and the wax can accumulate causing a blockage. It's only a problem when the ear canal is completely or almost completely blocked. In this situation, a loss of hearing is noticed. The wax can be removed by your physician or audiologist. It is not a good idea to try to remove wax yourself. You could cause damage to your ear canal or eardrum.

## Otitis Media

In the middle ear behind the eardrum, the most common problem is a build-up of fluid. This can occur if you have a cold, upper respiratory infection or severe allergies. Due to inflammation, the *Eustachian tube* can become blocked. This tube is a conduit that runs between the middle ear and back of the upper throat and usually aerates and drains the middle ear space. During a cold, unwanted fluids can fill the middle ear, preventing normal conductance of sound and creating a mild hearing loss. This problem often resolves on its own, but can sometimes require medical treatment, especially if infection is involved.

In cases of chronic, long-term middle ear infection, more serious complications can occur. Severe middle ear infection with extreme pressure and blocked Eustachian tubes can cause the eardrum to rupture. Chronic infections over time can cause defects in the *ossicular chain* and/or the development of a growth called a cholesteatoma. A *cholesteatoma* is an abnormal growth of skin behind the eardrum which forms a foul smelling pouch. Over time, it can destroy middle ear bones and even spread into the inner ear or brain. These conditions require medical treatment and should not be ignored. Hearing loss will accompany these conditions, but may be at least partially correctable through surgery.

## Otosclerosis

This is a condition in which an abnormal bony growth develops in the middle ear, particularly around the footplate of the stapes bone. As you learned, the stapes is the bone that transmits the sound energy to the inner ear. In otosclerosis, the bony growth accumulates around the footplate of the stapes at the *oval window* of the cochlea, interfering with its back-and-forth movement and thus transmission of energy to the inner ear. This is a gradual process that takes place over a number of years, causing a progressive loss of hearing. It usually occurs in one ear at a time. The diagnosis of otosclerosis is based on a particular pattern of results found on a thorough hearing evaluation. A surgical procedure called a *stapedectomy* can be very successful in correcting otosclerosis. During this procedure, the stapes bone is broken away from the incus and the bony growth around the oval window is cleared away. Then, a prosthesis is connected to the incus and sealed around the oval window, replacing the function of the stapes bone and restoring hearing.

Tinnitus can develop with any type of conductive hearing loss. Even something as benign as wax build-up can cause the perception of tinnitus. If a conductive hearing loss is the cause, the tinnitus will often be alleviated by removal or treatment of the problem causing the hearing loss.

## Sensorineural Hearing Loss

Sensorineural hearing loss is any hearing loss due to dysfunction of the inner ear, auditory nerve or neural pathways. Sometimes these are referred to generically as "nerve losses." Most sensorineural hearing losses, however, are caused by loss of sensory hair cells in the cochlea. This kind of hearing loss is very common because loss of hair cells occurs naturally with age. When the loss is determined to be due to aging, it's called *presbycusis*. However, loss of hair cells can also be caused by loud noise, by some medications, and by illness. Most sensorineural hearing losses are irreversible. The following is a description of some of the most common types of sensorineural hearing loss.

## Congenital Hearing Loss

When someone is born with a hearing loss it's called *congenital*. These can be due to either hereditary factors or something that occurred in the womb. Congenital hearing losses can range from mild to profound. The profound cases are more quickly identified because the infant doesn't respond to sound at all. Milder cases can take years to identify, especially if mild enough to allow a child to develop speech and language normally. Some congenital hearing losses are mild at birth, but progress to more severe hearing loss over time.

## Presbycusis

As stated earlier, this is the type of hearing loss most of us will develop with age. With the passing of each year of our life, we lose approximately 0.5% of our hair cells. Therefore, by the time we reach age 60, we've lost about 30% of our hair cells. So it's no wonder that the prevalence of hearing loss increases dramatically over the age of 60 years. The aging process can also cause deterioration of other neural structures, beyond the level of the hair cells. Presbycusis develops slowly over time, and varies in degree across individuals, from mild to severe. There's a definite pattern in cases of presbycusis: the high frequencies (high pitches) will be affected first.

At this point in your reading, it would be a good idea to learn about the *audiogram*. An audiogram (shown below) is a graphical representation of hearing as noted on a hearing test. The O's represent the thresholds of hearing for the right ear; X's represent the left ear. A threshold is the softest sound one can hear on the test. The audiogram shows hearing thresholds for a range of frequency (or pitch) from low (250 Hz) to high (8000 Hz). Frequency (Hz) is labeled across the top of the chart while intensity in *decibels* (dB) is along the side. For the individual represented in Figure 7-2 diagnosed with presbycusis, as sound gets higher in frequency, it needs to be more intense for him to hear.

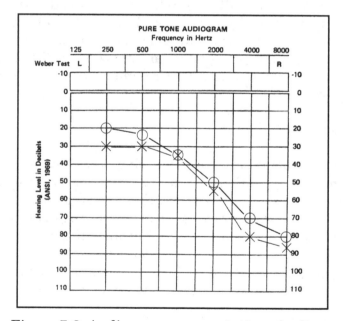

Figure 7-2: Audiogram representation of a diagnosis of presbycusis

People with presbycusis (high frequency hearing loss) will report that they can usually <u>hear</u> someone talking but they often <u>misunderstand</u> what's being said. This is because they can hear the low frequency components of a person's voice, but they miss the high frequency consonant sounds which carry most of the information for the clarity of speech. The problem of understanding is worse in conditions of background noise because the noise contains a lot of low frequency energy that serves to cover up the softer high frequency sounds. People with presbycusis often develop tinnitus gradually over time along with the hearing loss. Hearing aids can help with both the hearing and the tinnitus.

## Noise-induced Hearing Loss

This type of hearing loss is also due to the loss of hair cells, but is not a natural process. In this case, the hair cells are damaged by the bombardment of high levels of noise. The degree of damage from noise exposure is dependent on several factors: the level of the noise; the duration of exposure; the type of noise (for example, impulse noise is more damaging than steady-state noise); and the individual "toughness" of the ear. In general, the louder the sound, the less time it will take to cause damage to the ear. However, you can take two individuals, expose them to the same amount of noise, and one may develop more hearing loss than the other. In other words, some people are more susceptible to noise-induced hearing loss than others. It's also important to note that the damage from noise exposure can occur gradually over a long period of time. It could take ten years of working in a noisy factory or playing in a rock band before any hearing loss is noticed. By that time, the irreversible damage is done.

A person with noise-induced hearing loss will complain of the same problems of misunderstanding words, and difficulty hearing in background noise. Tinnitus is quite common in cases of noise-induced hearing loss, and can sometimes be initiated by a single exposure to very loud sound.

The typical noise-induced audiogram will resemble that of presbycusis in that the high frequencies will be most affected. However, in the case of noise-induced hearing loss (at least in the early stages), there will usually be a slight improvement in hearing at about 8000 Hz. The greatest hearing loss is usually at the frequency of 4000 Hz. The "4000 Hz notch" is a distinguishing feature of hearing loss caused by noise. This simply means there can be some recovery (improved hearing) above 4000 Hz. This is illustrated in Figure 7-3 on the next page.

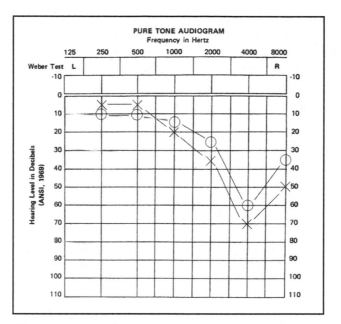

Figure 7-3: Audiogram representation of noise-induced hearing loss with a "notch" at 4,000 Hz.

## Ménière's Disease

Although Ménière's disease is not nearly as common as presbycusis or noise-induced hearing loss, it is important to the subject of this book because one of the main symptoms of this disease is a low-pitched roaring type of tinnitus. People with Ménière's disease experience recurring episodes of vertigo or dizziness, roaring tinnitus, a feeling of fullness in the ear, and hearing loss. Ménière's disease is thought to be caused by an overproduction and/or poor absorption of the fluid that surrounds the organ of Corti and hairs cells. It's thought that an excess of this *endolymphatic fluid,* creates increased pressure within the cochlea causing the hearing loss, tinnitus, and feeling of fullness in the ear. The same fluid also fills the part of the inner ear responsible for balance where increased pressure causes vertigo accompanied by nausea and vomiting.

Ménière's disease usually occurs in only one ear. However, in some people, the other ear may eventually also become affected. The attacks of vertigo and nausea are most severe in the early stages of the disease, and over time tend to become less severe. On the other hand, the hearing loss and tinnitus may become progressively worse over time. Treatment may include drug therapy, modification in diet and/or surgery in cases of continued incapacitating vertigo.

## Sudden Hearing Loss

Sudden sensorineural hearing loss can be caused by drugs, trauma or illness. Often, the cause is unknown. In these cases, the term *sudden idiopathic sensorineural hearing loss* is used. A common report is that upon wakening in the morning, the person first notices a ringing in one ear along with a feeling of fullness or a feeling of the ear being plugged. Sometimes people will also experience dizziness at the time of the sudden loss. The hearing loss is almost always in one ear, and usually severe. If medical attention is sought immediately, treatment with steroid drugs can help in some of these cases. However, if days or weeks go by, treatment is usually ineffective. In most cases, the dizziness subsides, but the hearing loss is permanent and tinnitus may continue.

## Tumor on the Auditory Nerve

A tumor on the eighth cranial nerve is another condition that can cause a variety of symptoms, including hearing loss, tinnitus and dizziness. The eighth cranial nerve is the nerve that sends both hearing and balance information to the brain. These tumors are benign and very slow growing. They're referred to by a variety of names including: vestibular schwannoma; acoustic neuroma; acoustic schwannoma; and eighth nerve tumor. The first symptoms are usually hearing loss and tinnitus in one ear. Other symptoms that may occur over time, and depending on the size and exact location of the tumor, include dizziness, loss of balance, facial numbness, weakness or tingling, and headache. Magnetic resonance imaging (MRI) is the gold standard for definitive diagnosis. Surgery is usually recommended to remove the tumor, but a period of watchful waiting may be recommended depending on the patient's age and overall health. The goal of surgery is to remove the tumor and if possible preserve the hearing, but often the hearing must be partially or totally sacrificed in the process. Tinnitus can continue following surgery regardless of whether or not the hearing was preserved.

## Effects of Hearing Loss on Communication and Quality of Life

At the beginning of this chapter, I spoke about the importance of hearing for both basic survival and as our means of communication and connection to others. In this section, I would like to expand on those ideas and discuss how hearing loss can affect our ability to communicate and our quality of life. The impact of hearing loss can vary greatly in relation to several factors: the degree of hearing impairment; the ability to understand speech; the management of the hearing loss; and the lifestyle of the individual.

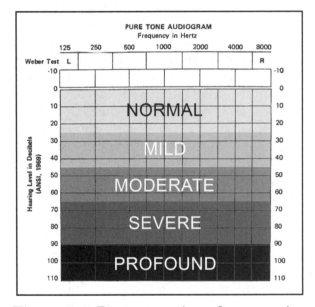

Figure 7-4: Representation of progressive degrees of hearing loss in decibels across the most important frequencies for understanding speech

We'll start with the degree of hearing loss. Regardless of the cause, hearing loss can be described as mild, moderate, severe or profound. Figure 7-4 shows the degree of hearing loss on an audiogram. This gets a little tricky because one can have a mild loss in some frequency ranges, while having a severe loss at other frequencies (as we discussed in the section on presbycusis). However, we can usually categorize the degree of hearing loss as an average across many frequencies, or describe it with a range of severity, (for example, mild-to-moderate loss). The degree of hearing loss is best expressed in decibels (dB HL) which are a measure of intensity shown along the left side of the audiogram. The HL after dB means Hearing Level, and provides a standardized reference to quantify the level.

## Mild hearing loss

If hearing thresholds are in the range of 25-45 dB HL, this is considered a mild loss, with normal hearing thresholds being in the range of 0 to 25 dB HL. People with a mild loss of hearing do quite well in face-to-face conversation, and in small groups. However, listening begins to require additional effort and concentration. Hearing from a distance, hearing in background noise and understanding softer voices becomes difficult. It seems that people are mumbling at times. Hearing aids might be recommended when the loss averages 30 dB HL or higher.

## Moderate hearing loss

If thresholds average 45 to 65 dB HL, the loss is considered to be moderate. With a moderate degree of impairment, normal conversational speech becomes difficult to hear. Since a normal conversational voice is about 50 dB HL, if your average hearing threshold is 45 dB HL, you'll hear the voice but it'll seem soft, and you'll have to really concentrate. If your average hearing threshold is 60 dB HL, you'll have trouble hearing most voices unless the person speaks louder than normal. You can imagine that the impact of a moderate loss is much more pronounced than the mild loss. Hearing aids are most definitely needed at this point. Without the assistance of hearing aids, the person with a moderate degree of hearing loss will be exhausted from the effort of listening. They'll tend to withdraw from conversation and social activities which can lead to social isolation and depression. The good news is most people with moderate hearing loss will function very well with hearing aids.

## Severe hearing loss

Hearing thresholds averaging 65 to 90 dB HL are considered to be in the severe range. At this level most conversation is inaudible. Without amplification you're cut off from others, severely limited in your ability to communicate. Hearing aids are required to restore some degree of audibility, but you'll need to supplement what you hear with visual cues. In most cases of severe hearing loss, there's distortion of speech even with the use of hearing aids. The hearing aids make sound more audible, but not necessarily clear. Imagine if you had a nice stereo system with a powerful amplifier, but you connected it to a pair of bad speakers; the result would be something like how the person with a severe hearing loss hears, even with the best hearing aids. Of course, without the hearing aids, the person would not hear much at all, so proper amplification is very much needed. In addition, the hearing-impaired person will need to make the most of other cues obtained by watching the speaker's lips, facial gestures, and body language (which we call *speechreading*—everybody does it, even with normal hearing). Knowing the context of the conversation is also very helpful. The brain will combine auditory and visual information, and relate it to knowledge of our language in the context of the situation in order to get the meaning of the message. Some people are better at this than others, and their success will depend on the situation (the complexity of the message, the distance from the speaker, the acoustics and lighting of the room, and so forth). Consequently, there's great variation in how much a person with severe loss will be able to understand in any one situation.

## Profound hearing loss

Hearing thresholds of 90 dB HL or greater are considered to be profound. Sometimes the term "deaf" is used for profound hearing loss. There are few sounds in our environment that are as loud as 90 dB HL, so this person lives in an essentially silent world. Hearing aids can provide some awareness of sound, but very little speech understanding. The person with a profound hearing loss is heavily reliant on visual cues, speechreading and sometimes s*ign language.*

If hearing aids are of little or no benefit, this person might be a candidate for a *cochlear implant.* A cochlear implant is a device that is implanted in the skull behind the ear, with an electrode which is placed into the cochlea. An external transmitter and processor, which looks something like a large hearing aid picks up sounds from the environment, transforms the sound into an electrical signal, and delivers that signal through the skin to the internal electrode. The electrical impulses stimulate the remaining nerve fibers in the inner ear which then sends messages to the brain. Although cochlear implants cannot restore normal hearing, they can be very beneficial to the profoundly hearing-impaired individual by restoring awareness of sound and surprisingly valuable speech information to nearly all recipients.

## Factors that Impact Hearing Loss

Having established the range of degree of hearing impairment from mild to profound, now let's look at other factors that have an affect on the impact of hearing loss.

1. The degree of hearing loss can vary across frequency.
As mentioned previously, you can have milder loss, or even normal hearing at some frequencies (pitches), and more severe loss at other frequencies. The most common situation is that the hearing is better in the low frequencies and poorer in the higher frequencies. If the low frequency hearing is good, but the high frequencies are moderately to severely impaired, you'll have no trouble hearing others speaking, but will often misunderstand the words. So, persons with high frequency hearing loss report that they hear, but don't understand. Good news again here—there are hearing aids that can amplify the high frequencies and allow low frequencies to pass through unaffected, effectively increasing the clarity of speech.

2. Speech understanding ability can vary regardless of the degree of hearing loss.
As part of the hearing evaluation, the audiologist will test your ability to understand words. This test will be performed at a comfortably loud level, so it's testing how well you can understand words once they're loud enough. For some people, once the volume is turned up, they understand clearly. For others, even with enough volume, the words are not clear. The speech understanding test is scored according to the percent of words correctly repeated, from 0 to 100%. Two people can have the same degree of hearing loss, but be very different in their ability to understand speech. For example, a person with a moderate hearing loss and excellent speech understanding (let's say 90%) will understand most speech with the use of hearing aids. On the other hand, a person with a moderate loss and only fair speech understanding (say 60%) will have a greater degree of disability and not perform as well with hearing aids.

3. <u>The hearing loss is either unilateral or bilateral</u>.
It's possible to have hearing loss in only one ear or a mild loss in one ear with a more severe loss in the other. This will obviously enter into the overall degree of impairment. Even if a person has one ear with perfectly normal hearing, a loss in the other ear will be noticeable. Of course, the impact of a unilateral hearing loss will vary according to degree. People with unilateral hearing loss will commonly report difficulty telling where sounds are coming from, along with increased difficulty in noisy situations.

4. <u>There are demands on listening</u>.
The impact of any degree of hearing loss will vary according to the demands placed on you for listening in your particular life situation. A mild hearing loss with good speech understanding may be hardly noticed by you if you live alone, are no longer working, and can turn up the volume on your TV and radio. On the other hand, that same mild hearing loss can have a huge impact on a court reporter who has to hear and record every word spoken in a courtroom. A hearing aid may be considered a necessity for an individual with high listening demands in their life, but more of an option for the person without many demands on their hearing. Of course, once the hearing loss gets beyond the mild category, the hearing aid is recommended for most, regardless of lifestyle.

5. <u>Management of the hearing loss is required</u>.
If the hearing loss is properly evaluated and recommendations for treatment are followed, the remaining hearing can be optimized and the impact of hearing loss can be minimized. Your willingness and motivation to optimize the use of hearing aids, visual cues, attention and focus, will aid in your overall ability to be a successful communicator regardless of your hearing loss. A positive attitude and good sense of humor can go a long way toward this goal. However, if not addressed and unmanaged, the hearing loss can have far-reaching detrimental effects on your quality of life. The obvious effect is on ability to communicate, but following the loss of communication comes a cascade of other consequences including:

**Social isolation:** When the effort required to engage in social situations exceeds the ability to enjoy those situations, you tend to draw away more and more, and can eventually become socially isolated.

**Effect on job and ability to work:** Unmanaged hearing loss can effect or prevent an individual from being able to perform on their job. This can lead to dissatisfaction on the parts of both the hearing-impaired person and their supervisor. The individual may feel they have no choice but to change jobs or retire. This situation is particularly unfortunate and unnecessary because of the existence of a law, the *Americans with Disabilities Act,* which protects the rights of individuals with hearing loss in the workplace. If your hearing loss is addressed, adequate accommodations must be put in place by your employer. Aids like amplified telephones or additional visual aids must be provided.

**Depression:** Difficulty in communicating, social isolation, or loss of employment can have a devastating effect on an individual's sense of well-being and interpersonal relationships; depression, stress and anxiety can result.

**Memory:** If you don't hear clearly, you certainly won't be able to remember what was said. This can be interpreted by others as a memory problem. It's a common misinterpretation of hearing loss among the elderly.

**Dementia:** Assessment of early dementia is often complicated or misdiagnosed due to the coexistence of hearing loss. It can be very difficult to sort out the effects of not being able to hear and socialize from the effects of dementia itself. It is also theorized that the loss of hearing, and consequent disconnect from the world, can hasten the progression of dementia.

These consequences may seem rather severe to you, but they're realistic outcomes of ignoring the existence of hearing loss. Of course, the point to be made here is that this doesn't need to happen! If diagnosed early and with proper treatment and follow-up, a hearing loss is quite manageable, and a very normal and successful life is possible for anyone with hearing loss. Hearing aids, although not able to restore normal hearing, can enable you to communicate well in most situations. The use of amplification (hearing aids) also helps to preserve speech understanding ability by continuing to provide stimulation to the auditory system. Amplification, along with additional conscious use of visual cues and contextual information, as mentioned previously, will help ensure that you stay active and connected in your world.

## Evaluation and Diagnosis of Hearing Loss

Now that you have some idea of the variation in the types and causes of hearing loss and the effects of hearing loss, you can appreciate the importance of a proper evaluation and diagnosis. Often, the earliest signs of hearing loss are very subtle: a slight ringing in the ear, difficulty hearing in background noise, having to ask people to repeat what they said a little more frequently. If you notice any of these symptoms, you should have a hearing evaluation. This first step sounds simple enough, but is often a hurdle for some people. Denial is a major factor in procrastination; it's natural to want to deny the fact that we're getting older, or that we may have a developed a dysfunction, no matter how mild. A typical strategy is to blame others for mumbling, which of course does not go over well with the people who are around you all the time and causes its own set of problems. So, the bottom line is, if you think you may have a hearing problem, you probably do and you should seek an evaluation.

In today's healthcare maze, it can be difficult to figure out where to start in seeking a hearing evaluation. Your primary care physician is always a good place to start. He or she can refer you to an audiologist for a hearing evaluation, or to an otologist or otolaryngologist for a medical evaluation of your ears. An audiologist is a healthcare provider who has a master's or doctoral degree in audiology. They practice in a variety of settings, including private audiology practices, speech and hearing centers, hospital clinics, and otolaryngology offices. An audiologist is uniquely trained in the evaluation and rehabilitation of hearing loss. They test hearing, diagnose the type and degree of hearing loss, recommend and dispense hearing aids, and provide follow-up and rehabilitation of hearing disorders. They are also trained to detect any underlying causes of hearing loss, and will refer you to a medical specialist if needed. An otologist is a medical doctor who specializes in the diagnosis and treatment of ear problems, including hearing loss. An otolaryngologist is a medical doctor who specializes in ear, nose and throat problems.

If you go to the medical specialist, they will order an audiological evaluation. Either way, you can be assured of having a thorough diagnostic hearing evaluation and proper recommendations. One word of caution here: do not go to a commercial store that sells hearing aids for your initial hearing evaluation, even if they are offering a "free hearing test." A store test will usually be a simple test for the purpose of fitting a hearing aid, not a diagnostic evaluation, and might miss an important underlying health condition. Be sure to be seen initially by an audiologist or otologist.

### Tips for Families, Friends and Co-Workers

People who live or work with a hearing-impaired person can help make communication easier for them. Here are a few tips to keep in mind before you start talking to someone with hearing loss.

**Get their attention.** Be sure the person knows you're addressing them and establish eye contact.

**Speak clearly at a normal loudness level.** Assuming the person is properly aided, yelling does not help. Speak in a clear, normal voice. Do not overly exaggerate your words, but don't talk too fast either. Sometimes it even helps to slow down, just a little.

**Establish the context of your message.** Be sure the person has an idea of what you're talking about, so they can listen within the context of a particular subject. It would be helpful for them to know, for example, if you're talking about the weather or about the state of your marriage. Your marriage might depend on it!

**Try not to talk with food in your mouth** (none of us do that anyway, right?) or with your hands in front of your lips. This makes speechreading difficult.

**Idealize your environment.** If you need to have an important conversation, move to a quiet area with good lighting so the person can get the clearest auditory and visual message.

**Rephrase.** If the person doesn't understand something you say, don't just repeat it louder; rephrase or use different words to express it.

**Above all, be patient and understanding.** In most cases, your friend or loved one is working hard to understand you. Imagine trying to hear with earplugs in your ears all the time; it might give you a little insight on what it's like to have a hearing loss. If you both make a little extra effort, communication does not have to be a problem.

### Hearing Loss and Tinnitus

By now, you must be wondering how tinnitus relates to all this information about hearing and hearing loss. After all, if you're reading this book, you or one of your loved ones is probably trying to deal with tinnitus. So in this last section, we'll look at the relationship between tinnitus and hearing loss.

There are a number of frequently asked questions about how tinnitus and hearing loss are related, including:

- Is the tinnitus caused by my hearing loss?
- Will the tinnitus make my hearing worse?
- If my hearing gets worse, will my tinnitus also get worse?
- Does the tinnitus interfere with my hearing?

When we look at factors such as severity of hearing loss, type and causes of hearing loss, or onset of hearing loss, tinnitus seems to be a free agent. Tinnitus can occur with any degree of hearing loss, any type of hearing loss, with any cause or type of onset. The severity of the tinnitus is not related to the severity of the hearing impairment. We occasionally see a person with normal hearing and tinnitus. However, in the vast majority of cases, tinnitus occurs with some type of hearing loss. Hearing scientists believe that tinnitus is due to some sort of change that has occurred within the auditory system. As you now know, the auditory system is complicated and this change can happen at many different levels within the system. Therefore, trying to tie the cause of the tinnitus to a particular event within the system is often futile. Having said that, if you have tinnitus, but have never had a hearing evaluation, you should get that hearing evaluation now. As mentioned earlier, tinnitus can sometimes be the first indication of hearing loss and any underlying medical issues should be ruled out.

Changes in hearing loss and changes in tinnitus also seem to occur independently of one another. Your tinnitus can increase or decrease without any change occurring in your hearing. Your hearing could get worse, but the tinnitus could remain unchanged, or even fade as you habituate to it. The message here is, don't spend time worrying about how your hearing and tinnitus might affect each other. You should always protect your hearing from extremely loud sound, such as loud concerts, power equipment, industrial noise, shooting guns, and so forth. But overprotection of hearing can become an obsession with some tinnitus patients because they're so worried about increasing the tinnitus. Use common sense and use earplugs when exposed to extremely loud noise, but not in everyday situations like driving or shopping.

The question of whether tinnitus interferes with hearing is an interesting one. We know that tinnitus does not actually change hearing thresholds. We can test a person's hearing on a day when their tinnitus is particularly bad, and then repeat the test on a better day and obtain the same hearing thresholds. However, the patient may tell us that it seems as if their hearing is worse on that loud tinnitus day.

The perception of increased hearing difficulty when tinnitus is disturbing is most likely due to difficulty in concentration and focus. Tinnitus can be very distracting and tends to call attention to itself, taking attention away from other sounds or listening tasks. Attention is an important factor in our ability to hear and process sound. When we're stressed or tired, from tinnitus and sleep deprivation, maintaining attention is even more difficult.

In some cases, tinnitus might be confused with sounds in our environment, such as crickets, birds or high-pitched alarm signals. Although most people will learn to recognize the difference between their tinnitus and real sounds, the similarities can initially be very disconcerting. In other cases, it may actually be that the tinnitus is masking some sounds. Some patients will say, "I found it difficult to hear them talking through my tinnitus."

## Summary

I hope that this chapter has provided you with some insight into the complexity of the auditory system and a framework in which to better understand your own hearing loss. The importance of proper evaluation and management of hearing loss and tinnitus should be clear in light of the impact hearing loss can have on your ability to communicate and the quality of your life. Armed with a thorough understanding of your hearing loss, you are in an excellent position to work with an audiologist or otologist who specializes in tinnitus and hearing. This person can provide you with assistive devices and strategies which will help to overcome the difficulties you may now be facing. I wish you success on your journey!

## Reference

Kochkin, S. (2005). MarkeTrak VII: Hearing Loss Population Tops 31 Million People, *The Hearing Review*, 12(7): 16-29.

# CHAPTER EIGHT

# Sleeping Better with Tinnitus

## Laurence McKenna, PhD and David Scott, PhD
*Royal National Throat, Nose & Ear Hospital, London*

---

**Dr. McKenna** has worked as a clinical psychologist at the Royal National Throat, Nose & Ear Hospital for the past 24 years. During this time he has been involved in the study of tinnitus and other audiological disorders and in the psychological management of patients with these problems. He is head of the team of psychologists working in Adult Audiological Medicine and is a member of the cochlear implant team. Other work at Guy's and St Thomas' Hospitals in London has included the assessment and management of patients with neurological disorders, medico-legal work, management of attempted suicide patients, cochlear implantation and sleep disorders. He is an honorary lecturer at the Ear Institute (UCL) and Visiting Fellow at the University of Bristol.

**Dr. Scott** has worked as a clinical psychologist at the Royal National Throat, Nose and Ear Hospital, London, since 2000. His primary clinical interest is tinnitus. He teaches at the Ear Institute, University College London, on the psychological management of tinnitus. He worked in a number of services in New Zealand including pediatric and cardiac/respiratory medicine before coming to the UK in 1998 where he worked in the mental healthcare of older adults before returning to his specialist interest in health psychology.

---

## Introduction

Much of the material weaved throughout this chapter will fit nicely with what you'll read in Chapter 5 of this book. For example, in that chapter you'll read about the cognitive behavioral model, the principles applicable to the role of "thinking" when trying to improve sleep, the distress related to tinnitus, the methods for identifying your thoughts about tinnitus and testing their accuracy—much of it easily applied to the problem of poor sleep. You'll see how you can test your thoughts by changing how you do things and be offered some questions to aid these reflections. And Chapter 5's reminder of the process of identifying and changing tinnitus-related safety behaviors will help you better understand this chapter.

## I Have Tinnitus. Will I Ever Get to Sleep?

In a word, yes. Whilst many people with tinnitus have trouble sleeping, most don't. There's no reason why you too can't sleep well. You might find it reassuring to know that most people who have tinnitus do not feel the need to attend tinnitus clinics since tinnitus doesn't play an important part in their lives. Nonetheless, a lot of people do struggle with their tinnitus and do seek professional help to learn to live with it.

About half of the patients we see in our tinnitus clinic say they sleep badly. This tells us that it is possible to sleep normally despite having tinnitus. In our experience it is usually not tinnitus itself that is the main factor in determining how well people sleep. Steven Wright, an American comedian and actor, said, "When I woke up this morning my girlfriend asked me, 'Did you sleep good?' I said 'No, I made a few mistakes.'" In this chapter we want to help you avoid some of the common mistakes on the journey to a good nights' sleep. Everyone suffers from episodes of bad sleep from time to time. It's easy to see how sleep might be disrupted when something significant happens in your life, like the onset of tinnitus. But why does the problem persist for some people and not for others? It may seem surprising, but those that say their tinnitus affects their sleep don't have different or easier tinnitus from those who do sleep well with tinnitus. This is good news because it means that you can have tinnitus and sleep well.

## A Model for Sleep

Dr. Alison Harvey, a psychologist, is one of the foremost researchers in the field of sleep. While at University of Oxford in England, she suggested that sleep problems persist over time because of thoughts and behavioral factors irrespective of what may have caused *insomnia* to develop initially. Her research led her to the conclusion that people don't sleep well because their minds are busy with worrying thoughts. These thoughts are stressful and so you'll become more aroused and awake. The stress leads you to focus your attention on your sleep and monitor it. As you monitor your sleep, your mind becomes busier and your perception of how much time you spend awake becomes distorted. Other difficulties also can seem more overwhelming than they actually are.

Whenever we're confronted with potential misfortune, we will usually try some strategies to prevent it happening or reduce the consequences if it does happen. Psychologists call these strategies "safety behaviors" because they're intended to keep us safe. Although safety behaviors can help us to feel better in the short term, over time they often keep the worries alive or even make them worse.

Our beliefs about how much sleep we need and what will happen if we don't get enough will influence how worried we become when we aren't sleeping well. For example, we might believe that a good nights' sleep is essential to be able to do our jobs well. Then when we have a disturbed night, we might fret about it, thinking we'll be unable to function at work the next day. These worrying thoughts can create more stress arousal, so making us more awake, cause us to monitor our sleep excessively, and then become even more stress-aroused. All this will probably ensure that the bad nights' sleep we feared does come about. Having one bad night can make us more anxious about the next night, and so on, so that a real sleep deficit can develop and persist even when the original cause of the insomnia is long gone. One of the most helpful things about Dr. Harvey's work on insomnia is the idea that poor sleep needs to be understood as a twenty-four hour process. The worry, stress, selective attention, monitoring and changes in behavior that occur at night can also be observed in the person during the daytime!

From these ideas Dr. Harvey proposed a cognitive behavioral model of sleep. This model certainly rings true when we talk to people who have poor sleep. Most people who suffer from insomnia say that it is a <u>busy mind</u> that keeps them awake rather than a <u>busy body</u>. The comedian Stephen Wright spoke about making a few mistakes when he tried to sleep. The cognitive behavioral model helps us to understand what these mistakes might be and gives us a clear direction for helping people. The principles that apply to other people with sleep problems also apply to people with tinnitus who sleep badly. When we help tinnitus patients with their sleep we therefore look to see what mistakes they may be making in terms of the worries they may have, the general beliefs they have about sleep, the stress arousal they experience, the monitoring they carry out and the safety behaviors they engage in. We work with our patients to help them identify where things are going wrong and to find a more helpful approach to sleep. In the remainder of this chapter we'll go into each of these cognitive behavioral ideas in more detail.

## Patterns of Sleep

To set the scene, let's begin with some general information about sleep. This will help provide a context for the other parts of the cognitive behavioral approach. There are a number of different schools of thought about sleep and particularly about the effects of lack of sleep. The information that we present here is derived from the work of psychologists and other researchers who have carried out careful experimental and clinical work with people who experience disturbed sleep.

### What Does Normal Sleep Look Like?

Fiona, one of our patients, developed sleep problems after the onset of her tinnitus. She had difficulty going to sleep, woke up several times a night and had trouble getting back to sleep. She felt exhausted the next day and believed she didn't function well. Like many other people, Fiona believed that a good night's sleep involved a straight eight hours of uninterrupted oblivion followed by refreshed and alert wakefulness throughout the day. Let us consider how well this idea matches what is known about sleep.

Our sleep changes with age, so what's normal when we're 5 years old will be different when we are 12 and different again when we are 40 and 70. Sleeping is more complex than simply falling asleep and waking in the morning. Our sleep consists of repeating cycles of *rapid eye movement* (REM) and non-REM sleep; the latter is divided into stages 1, 2, 3, and 4, corresponding to increasing depth of sleep where 1 represents light sleep and 4 represents deep sleep. The cycles of REM and non-REM sleep last approximately 90 minutes but can vary normally from 70 to 120 minutes. This cycle repeats about four or five times a night in young adults. Babies generally have more REM sleep than adults and spend more time asleep overall than adults. It comes as a surprise to many people to learn that we routinely wake in the night as part of the pattern of sleep described above. As we age we have less deep sleep (stage 4) and tend to wake more often. The first episode of waking occurs after two to three hours of sleep. If all is well, we may be unaware of these awakenings and just roll over and return to sleep. After the first awakening, we get more REM sleep and less deep sleep for the remainder of the night. Young people may wake twice a night but older adults may wake as often as nine times a night. Older adults often experience their sleep as being light and fragmented in nature.

When we're asleep, we're not in a state of simple oblivion. We've seen that there are several different stages, or types, of sleep. Most dreaming takes place during REM sleep. During this time the mind is quite busy but the body tends to be still. In contrast, in some non-REM sleep the body moves around more and the mind is less busy. Sometimes it's difficult for us to tell when we're asleep. A person can go on thinking about things even when in stage two sleep. Although it's common for most people to get between seven and nine hours sleep a night, there's significant variation between people. Some manage well on only four hours and others prefer ten. Older people tend to sleep less at night but they also nap more during the daytime and when the total amount of sleep they get over a 24-hour period is taken into account, it seems to be the case that the amount of sleep we get from middle age to later life is relatively stable.

Just as the amount of sleep required varies from person to person, it also differs from night to night for each of us. In addition to different sleep stages there's a daily biorhythm, with different stages, through which we pass. At certain stages within this rhythm, we feel sleepy and tend to function poorly (such as in the early hours of the morning and again in mid-afternoon) and at other times we feel awake and function well. The concept of the "siesta" nicely allows for these normal dips in arousal. These fluctuations in levels of arousal in the daytime occur even if we've slept well. So we can see that sleep is complex and a normal night's sleep involves light and deep sleep, dreaming, thinking, waking as well as periods of stillness. During the day we also experience different levels of alertness naturally. The ideas held by our patient, Fiona, therefore did not correspond well with what we know about a normal night's sleep and how we naturally feel during the day.

## Why do we Sleep?

Fiona believed that good sleep every night was essential to good health and day-to-day functioning. This is a belief that she shared with many other people. It's also widely known that deliberately depriving people of sleep for extended periods has been used as a form of torture. Some people believe that a lack of sleep will have similar effects to torture, possibly leading to insanity. Surprisingly, despite spending a third of our lives asleep, the purpose of sleep is unclear. There are a number of theories as to why we sleep but none of them is fully supported by the available research evidence. Although most of us feel bad if we have not slept well, the actual effects of sleep loss are not so clear. Very careful studies of people who complain of poor sleep suggest that they have a similar range of intellectual functioning the next day as people who have slept well. Studies of poor sleepers' physical status have also led researchers to question how much actual harm is caused by disturbed sleep. Some studies even suggest that when given the opportunity to sleep, poor sleepers don't fall asleep any quicker than people who have slept well. This suggests that the poor sleepers' tiredness does not translate into real sleepiness. When people have deliberately stayed awake, with no sleep at all for several days and nights, they still seem able to do most tasks reasonably well and appear reasonably healthy. Afterwards, when permitted to sleep, they do so for only slightly longer than they would usually.

These observations raise questions about whether sleep loss itself (as distinct from the stress involved in not sleeping) actually results in any loss of ability to function normally. Recent research suggests that although prolonged periods without any sleep do not have a significant effect on a person's ability to perform logical tasks. The research, however, suggests that sustained sleep loss does disrupt the ability to perform tasks that require more innovative, creative or "executive" thinking where the solutions to a problem are not obvious and where there may be false trails or irrelevant information to be avoided. It is important to remember, however, that most people's poor sleep or insomnia does not involve total sleep loss for days; usually poor sleepers do get some sleep. It's therefore not clear whether their executive thinking is affected.

From the above, it should be clear that sleep research is a field where findings vary, but taken as a whole, it is reasonable to conclude that while sleep loss does have some effects on people's ability to function, these effects are less than many people suppose. This is particularly true when the variations in functioning associated with the daily biorhythm are taken in to account. This conclusion stands in contrast with the everyday beliefs about sleep that many people hold, and also against some studies that suggest that poor sleep leads to ill health. Careful thought needs to be given to these differences. One part of the explanation may have to do with stress. The people who stayed awake for days and nights on end volunteered for the experience and were not highly stressed by it. Very often poor sleep results from high stress levels and it may be that ill health results from this, or from the stresses that arise from people's efforts to cope with sleep difficulties, rather than the lack of sleep alone.

## Worrying

We all worry at times, but some of us worry a lot. Many people believe worrying can be useful, such as preventing bad things from happening, enhancing coping, problem solving and being prepared. On the flip-side, worry increases your sensitivity to threat-related information. This means that you will become more aware of the things that you worry about and may worry even more about them. So a vicious circle develops. Bedtime may offer us an opportunity to reflect on the cares of the day. Once again the busy mind can set-up a system for keeping us awake.

## The Importance of Thinking

At the heart of the cognitive behavioral model is the idea that how you think about things determines how you feel. Some people find this a little difficult to accept because they're convinced that tinnitus is the thing that's making them feel bad and stopping them from sleeping. The evidence indicates that when tinnitus is experienced as very distressing, the distress is associated with worrying about tinnitus more than with how loud the tinnitus is or what it sounds like. Remember that we said that many people who are very distressed by tinnitus sleep well. Researchers have found that thinking, or cognitive processes, are ten times more likely than physical irritations or symptoms to be cited by insomniacs as the main reason for poor sleep. This places thinking at the heart of most sleep problems.

It's helpful to know that how we think about things is not set in stone. Different people might think about the same thing in different ways and one person might think about something in different ways at different times. The experience of thinking while lying awake in the middle of the night provides an excellent example of this. At that time, problems often seem overwhelming and we can feel really bad about them. Yet, when we think about the same problem the next day, it can seem more manageable and we may feel more optimistic. The problem is the same. It may be a real and difficult issue for us, but in the night our thoughts about it have become overly negative and as result, our feelings about the problem have changed. When we're feeling stressed our thinking changes and can become distorted during the day as well as at night. We can all too quickly fall into a pattern of unhelpful thinking so that we feel low or anxious which in turn can make us more likely to think in an unhelpful or negative way. When tinnitus or sleep becomes involved in this sort of vicious cycle of unhelpful thinking and emotional distress, we suffer more.

Remember that our patient, Fiona, believed that her tinnitus was preventing her from sleeping. When she reflected on the matter, however, she was able to recognize that as she laid tossing and turning unable to sleep, her head was full of thoughts. When discussing her previous night's sleep with us, she said that uppermost in her mind was the idea that she wasn't getting enough sleep and she'd be too tired to be efficient in an important business meeting the next day. She also thought that she would be too tired to make her usual visit to the gym and believed that because this was a repeating pattern she was slowly gaining weight.

Another worrying idea for Fiona was that without adequate sleep she would become so fatigued that she'd end up having a nervous breakdown. She also believed that there was no escape from her tinnitus. When she woke in the morning she felt tired and drained of energy and as a consequence was convinced that her poor sleep was indeed having a very bad effect on her. These thoughts reflected her general beliefs about sleep but they were focused on the particular events of the day and on the likely consequences for her as an individual. It's easy to see that while these thoughts raced around her mind, she was going to find it very difficult to sleep. If Fiona had been able to appraise her situation differently, without expecting the worst with respect to her health and work, then she'd have been more likely to relax when in bed and increase her chances of falling asleep.

For Fiona, who is typical of many people who are not sleeping well, it's a busy mind, particularly one full of worrying thoughts, that was the central factor in maintaining poor sleep. This pattern of overly negative, distorted thinking about sleep and tinnitus increases poor sleep and awareness of tinnitus. Let's think about this suffering in a little more detail.

## Changes in Mood and Stress Arousal

To briefly summarize some of the key points from Chapter 5, Fiona's pattern of overly negative, unhelpful thinking led to her feeling of anxiety about her sleep and inability to cope with disturbed sleep, so she felt very low in her mood when she considered putting on weight. Anxiety and depression are common among our tinnitus patients and particularly among those who complain of sleep problems. We believe this is because people attach such importance to sleep and (wrongly) conclude that they'll suffer disastrous consequences if they lose some sleep.

Worrying thoughts can also be a source of stress and can have physical effects on our bodies. This increase in physical arousal can make it more difficult to sleep. Fiona felt very tense and experienced a racing heart. This led to a vicious cycle between her negative thoughts and physical symptoms of stress arousal.

## Focusing of Attention

When we feel threatened in some way, for example, by an external danger or by the possibility of not coping well at work because of poor sleep, we naturally focus our attention on the threat. Keeping an eye on something that poses a danger makes sense from a survival point of view. Our focus becomes evermore narrow the greater the perceived threat. This can mean that non-threatening things tend to be ignored so that more resources can be devoted to monitoring the threat. If you believe that tinnitus poses a threat to your sleep, you may focus your attention on it very selectively such that your awareness of the tinnitus increases. You may also carefully monitor your tinnitus by checking to see if it's louder than the bedside noise generator or to see if it has changed in tone. As your awareness of tinnitus increases by selective attention and monitoring, you may conclude that your belief that tinnitus is a very threatening problem is correct.

When we sleep poorly, we selectively attend to and monitor our sleep and the problems we anticipate from not sleeping well. Just as tinnitus becomes more noticeable the more we attend to and monitor it, sleep also becomes more difficult as we focus on it. Our patients typically check the clock repeatedly during the night to see how long they've been awake or how many more hours of tossing and turning they'll have to endure before morning. They monitor their body for any signs of sleepiness (muscles relaxing, feeling of drifting off) or wakefulness (heart pounding, tight muscles). On waking, people tend to monitor their bodies for signs of poor sleep such as tiredness, or check the clock to see how much sleep they got. During the day they may check for signs of fatigue and critically examine their work performance, functioning and mood for the effects of sleep loss. When we look hard for something, we will often find it and it's common for people to attribute to poor sleep the benign and normal fluctuations in arousal that occur to all of us in the day. Again, the monitoring tends to feed the worry and a vicious cycle is created.

### Changes in Perception

A particularly interesting part of Dr. Harvey's model of insomnia is the suggestion that people who suffer from insomnia experience a change in their perception of how much (or little) they sleep. She suggests that poor sleepers overestimate how long it takes to fall asleep and underestimate the total amount of sleep they get. It's likely that this "distortion" of perception results from the monitoring discussed above. It also results from the fact that the period just prior to onset of sleep and the moment of sleep itself are elusive and so we don't have a clear memory of these events. Further, if we're awake for a long time, there's greater chance for our time estimations to be subject to errors of judgment, particularly if we're stressed. We also think that selective attention and monitoring, particularly when we're already stressed, can lead to a similar distortion in our perception of tinnitus. This might explain why some people describe tinnitus as sounding like a "jack hammer," "jet plane" or "steam train." These changes in perception may strengthen worrying thoughts about tinnitus, sleep and the consequences of lack of sleep.

### Changes in Behavior

When confronted with a danger, real or imagined, we naturally try do something to avert the crisis. All children will be familiar with the scary monster under the bed. As adults, we know there's nothing there, but a child's vivid imagination will interpret that odd sound or the shape of a shadow as conclusive evidence there really is a seriously nasty monster in the room. Adults are prone to the same errors of judgment when it comes to danger (although most us no longer worry about monsters) and such misinterpretations of the degree of threat are likely to be greatest when we're already under stress. Common errors include overestimating the likelihood of something bad happening, or that it will be more threatening than is really the case, or underestimate the resources available to help us cope with it. We may misinterpret the evidence we have available or perhaps disregard or dismiss evidence that our fears are not well-founded. We all know how problems can appear magnified when we think about them in the middle of the night, yet often seem more manageable during the middle of the day. If our view of a problem is based upon "middle of the night" thinking and we act to keep safe in line with that view, then the safety behaviors we employ to do this may hinder us from seeing the problem from the perspective of "middle of the day" thinking.

Fiona believed that being in a quiet environment would result in her tinnitus becoming more intrusive and possibly overwhelming her. There was always some background sound wherever she went that was loud enough to compete with her tinnitus. The bedroom became a place of dread for her and she acted to keep safe by having the television on whenever she got into bed. By keeping herself safe with background sound she stopped herself from finding out whether a quieter environment would result in her tinnitus overwhelming her. Her anxieties were therefore kept alive by her behavior. Television programs and commercials aren't intended to put you to sleep, so not surprisingly, Fiona's reliance on the television actually kept her awake.

Nocturnal safety behaviors, such as Fiona's use of television, tend to interfere with the regularity of the sleep cycle, with getting to sleep, and provoke more thinking activity. Poor sleepers often use a number of safety behaviors in the day that have the effect of increasing daytime sleepiness, make the day less pleasant or more boring than it needs to be, and increases preoccupation with sleep. For example, Fiona's daytime safety behavior involved doing less than she'd normally do because she had a poor night's sleep.

## How Do I Make Things Better?

We've made the point that there's a considerable variation in how much sleep each of us requires and that our sleep can vary naturally from night to night. Another well-observed variation is that people with sleep problems often have a distorted perception of how long it takes them to get to sleep and how much sleep they get. This is not to say that real deficits in sleep do not occur. The more often we go around the vicious cycle of worrying thoughts, stress, selective attention and monitoring, distorted perception and changing our behavior, then greater the chance that our sleep will deteriorate to some extent.

To obtain a reasonably accurate picture of our patients' sleep, we ask them to quickly note in a diary at breakfast time answers to the following questions:

- What time did you go to bed?
- What time did you turn off the lights?
- How long did it take you to fall asleep?
- How many times did you awaken in the night?
- For how long were you awake in the night?
- What time did you finally wake up?
- What time did you get out of bed?
- What was the quality of your sleep (marks out of 10)?
- How long (if at all) did you nap in the day?

In the evening we ask them to rate how well they functioned during the day (marks out of 10). We caution our patients against watching the clock to obtain this information as a guess will often be accurate to within ten minutes or so and that's good enough. We examine the data using a computer spreadsheet which helps to do some arithmetic and allows us to generate some useful charts, but we can generally see the pattern of someone's sleep and identify key problem areas just by looking at the diary. We're interested in how long someone has spent in bed, at what time of day/night they're in bed, how much sleep they get, and whether the problem with their sleep occurs mainly at the beginning of the night, in returning to sleep in the middle of the night or in the morning. Keeping a diary of sleep in this way can also help you keep a track of the progress you make when you set about resolving your sleep problems. Very often, we find that in recording sleep in this structured way, many of our patients discover they're getting a little more sleep than they had believed. The same thing has been noticed in sleep laboratories where an *electroencephalograph* (EEG) of a patient's brainwaves during sleep often reveal that they're sleeping longer than they thought they were.

## Expectations for Sleep

If your sleep is poor, there are a number of changes you can make to improve it. It's helpful to understand what normal sleep consists of and to examine your beliefs about sleep so that you have realistic expectations about your sleep. For example, many of our tinnitus patients are reassured to know that it is normal to wake up during the night. Some of them blame tinnitus for waking them and are relieved to learn that their awakenings actually correspond to the normal night time awakenings.

## Changing Your Worrying Thoughts about Sleep and Tinnitus

Generally, people who have problems sleeping are preoccupied by thoughts about falling asleep quickly and obtaining as much sleep as possible. These thoughts are often accompanied by other worries about the consequences of not getting sufficient sleep such as:

- decline in physical or mental health;
- inability to cope with the day ahead; and
- unresolved issues from the day before or longstanding concerns.

Most of us tend to worry about issues that we have not had time to think about sufficiently during the day. We might lie awake reflecting upon pleasant things or plan a new project or activity. Although positive in character, these thoughts can also keep us awake. Common thoughts about tinnitus might include:

- My tinnitus wakes me up.
- I can never get away from my tinnitus.
- I can never get tinnitus out of my mind.
- My tinnitus has affected my brain and ability to think.
- Life will never be the same again.
- I'll never get any peace and quiet.
- I can't enjoy things now.
- I can't do normal things, like sleep, anymore.
- I must avoid silence.
- Other people don't understand.
- It's not fair that this has happened to me.

In order to get at the heart of the matter it's sometimes necessary to "ladder" your thoughts. This involves writing down an idea that went through your mind and then asking yourself what the implication of that idea is. For example, if the first idea that you write down is "my tinnitus will never go away" or "I will never get to sleep," then it's useful to ask "What does this mean for me?" When Fiona did this exercise, the idea that first came to her head was, "I can't get away from this tinnitus." When she asked herself what the implication of this was she realized she also had the thought that, "I'll feel tired tomorrow and be unable to cope well." The implication of this for her was, "I'll fall behind in my work." The implication of this was, "I'll have to work harder and I'll get more and more tired and I'll still not be able to sleep." This implied that, "I'll become worn down by fatigue and eventually have a nervous breakdown!" In this way, Fiona built a "ladder" of her thoughts and identified the ideas that were causing her distress and that she needed to work on. It's not surprising that she found it hard to sleep with all these worrying ideas going through her mind. We find it helpful to remind our patients that our thoughts and actions concerning sleep in the daytime can be just as important as what happens at night.

Once you've identified your thoughts about sleep or tinnitus, the next step is to work out if they're accurate or the result of "middle of the night" or stressed thought processes. As cognitive therapists, we believe that our thoughts about a situation will have a big influence on how we feel. By changing the way we think about a situation, we can change how we feel. Thoughts can be correct, incorrect or only partially correct. It is important to consider that beliefs about a situation may not be correct even if they appear to be compelling at the time. It can be helpful to approach any investigations into the accuracy of our thoughts in the same way that a scientist investigates hypotheses that need to be tested. Changing how you think might come about as a result of careful reflection on the situation or it may be that you have to test your thoughts by changing how you do things. The essence of this approach is to consider what information or evidence you have that supports your worrying idea and what information you have that either contradicts the idea or supports an alternative perspective. Usually, we see other people's problems in a different light from our own, so it may be worthwhile considering what you might say to a friend who came to you for advice with the same worrying thoughts. Even if we recognize that our friend has a problem, we tend to see the problem in less serious terms and have greater confidence in their ability to cope with the situation than in our own. A variation on this theme is to consider what you might say or think about the situation if you were feeling less stressed. By taking a more objective view of the situation, the problem can become more manageable.

When Fiona recognized her worrying beliefs that she'd be tired and unable to cope well the next day and that this would lead to her falling behind on her work, she set about identifying the available evidence for and against these thoughts. We pointed out to her that these thoughts were about the future and therefore, by definition, she couldn't have any actual evidence to support them. However, this was not the first time she had experienced these thoughts so she could refer to evidence from previous occasions. When she carefully considered the previous occasions, Fiona remembered feeling tired during the day and that things had been a struggle, but she also recalled getting the essential things done and, to that extent, coping with the day. She also considered what she'd say to a friend who had not slept well and was feeling tired. She realized that she would convey her confidence in her friend's ability to cope with the day in spite of fatigue. Fiona then appreciated that she was able to cope with situations as well as her friend did. These reflections allowed her to feel less anxious about the day ahead.

As she went through the following day, Fiona kept a note on how she felt and how she performed at work. She felt very tired getting up in the morning and initially she took this as evidence of how bad she had slept the night before. But then she remembered that most people do feel sluggish on waking and that her fatigue was not all due to lack of sleep. She also discovered that she felt less tired as the morning went on. Fiona noted that despite an element of fatigue, she managed her essential duties that day. She realized that she worked at a slightly less frantic pace than usual because she deliberately didn't do a few things. By recording her real life observations, Fiona's anxiety about lack of sleep was further reduced. The diary of her activities and physical state provided her with evidence about what actually happens when she doesn't sleep well as opposed to what she thought happened. This evidence was then available to her the next time she didn't sleep well. Just being less anxious helped her mind to be less busy and less focused on her tinnitus and sleep which led to her sleeping better.

A great deal of unhelpful thinking can be addressed in the way Fiona addressed her worries about sleep. These techniques can help you to weaken or break the hold that negative thinking may have over you. The aim is not simply to think positive thoughts or, like Monty Python, to "look on the bright side." Rather, the point is to realize that there are different ways of understanding a situation and that the very worrying one that you assume to be right, may not be the one that is best supported by the evidence. It's not about absolutes or "black and white" thinking, but rather recognizing that there are shades of grey. The result will be less distress, less arousal and less focus on tinnitus.

## Changing Your Safety Behaviors

We've made the point that most people will seek to protect themselves from danger. When the threat is real, then protecting yourself has genuine survival value. When your perception of threat arises from very stressed or "middle of the night" thinking, however, then trying to keep safe can stop you finding out the real extent of the danger, and your worries will be kept alive or even made worse. Just as important as changing the way we think about sleep is changing sleep-related safety behaviors. Our safety behaviors are always linked to worrying thoughts so it is useful to consider the predictions we're making about what will happen if we don't sleep well. The predicted problems can be related to concrete consequences such as what we have to do at work or may be concerned with how we might feel if we don't sleep, such as feeling extremely anxious or tired. We can then identify our particular safety behaviors by asking ourselves what it is that we do to keep safe from these predictable problems.

Common sleep-related safety behaviors include:

- sleeping late in the morning (especially on the weekend);
- sleeping during the day;
- going to bed early;
- making plans for the next day at bedtime or in bed;
- exercising late in the day;
- watching television or reading in bed;
- telling yourself to stop worrying;
- telling yourself "I must go to sleep now;"
- taking the day easy;
- skipping exercise;
- canceling appointments;
- going to bed at a time determined by when you get up

- rather than when you feel ready to sleep;
- making plans for the day based on how much sleep you've had;
- making plans for catching-up on sleep.

Safety behaviors such as these interfere with the regularity of the sleep cycle and with getting to sleep. They provoke more thinking, exacerbate daytime sleepiness, contribute to the day being unpleasant or boring, and increase preoccupation with sleep. So you can see that the safety behaviors that are intended to help often have the opposite effect by contributing to many of the negative outcomes predicted. Safety behaviors also stop us from finding out that our thoughts are unrealistic and unhelpful. Once you have identified your worrying ideas about sleep and tinnitus and the safety behaviors you've put in place to prevent these bad things from happening, it's time to try doing things differently. Work out what you could do differently that would test your worrying idea. This might involve doing something in another way or perhaps not doing something that you would usually do. Once you've decided what to change, make a prediction about what will happen when you do so. Then try things out and note exactly what does happen and consider what the outcome means for your original worrying idea.

Remember that Fiona kept her television on when in bed in order to provide background noise. This was because she believed that being in a quiet environment would result in her tinnitus becoming intrusive and overwhelming. By keeping herself safe through the use of her television, Fiona prevented herself from finding out whether a quieter environment would actually result in her tinnitus overwhelming her. The use of the television also made her sleep worse. She agreed to test her anxious thought by not having the television on in her bedroom. She predicted that her tinnitus would be very loud, that she would get no sleep and be highly anxious. She also decided that she would not actively try to sleep, but would just see what happened. On the first night, Fiona was more aware of her tinnitus and did feel anxious for a long time but then, in spite of not trying to sleep, she did fall asleep. She gradually discovered over subsequent nights that she was less worried about the lack of the television and the impact on her sleep and soon she was sleeping better without the television than when she used if regularly. Fiona's belief that she'd be overwhelmed by anxiety unless she avoided tinnitus through constant noise was disproved. As a consequence of this experiment, she felt much more in control.

Fiona then tested another of her safety behaviors. She was anxious that she would be unable to do all the things she needed to do, or do them as well as she thought she had to, if she didn't sleep well. To cope with this anxiety, she kept herself safe by focusing only on the "important" things and ceased activities that seemed to her to be less vital such as going to the gym and seeing her friends. She believed that saving her energy for the important activities would help her get through the day and result in her being less tired. By avoiding the other activities, Fiona prevented herself from discovering that she could manage a full day on the sleep she was having and therefore she remained worried about this aspect of her sleep. The loss of exercise also made things worse because, contrary to her expectation, exercise made her feel more lively and less tired. Many people reduce what they do during the day after they've slept badly. Fiona cut out the things she regarded as less important (although they were also the activities that maintained her physical and mental well-being and provided a balance to the work-related stresses of her life). However, many people reduce important tasks for fear that they'll fail at them and restrict themselves to mundane and routine tasks. Doing this can make the day more tedious, leave us feeling frustrated and stressed because we are failing to fulfill our responsibilities. These worries and pressures can in turn contribute to us sleeping more poorly and so a vicious cycle is created.

## Good Sleep Hygiene

If the *Cognitive Behaviorial Therapy* (CBT) approach is not practical for you, for one reason or another, then there are a number of routines around sleeping and the bedroom that you can think about and try to improve.

## Reducing Stress

We can lower our level of physical and mental arousal associated with stress by using relaxation techniques. Clearly, the more aroused you are, the less likely you are to fall asleep. So it follows that greater relaxation, and with it lower levels of stress arousal, will promote the onset of sleep. Some of our patients also find that when they're relaxed, they experience their tinnitus as being less intrusive. Relaxation therapy techniques should be distinguished from other activities usually associated with relaxation, such as watching television or reading, in which we may be physically passive but are often aroused or stimulated mentally. Relaxing effectively isn't just a matter of lying down and doing nothing. It's an active process and a skilled set of techniques that require daily practice to become competent in. Most of our patients find it a pleasant process that takes no more than about 20 to 30 minutes a day. We use *progressive muscle relaxation techniques* in which each muscle group in the body is tensed and relaxed in turn. This process can enable you to develop your awareness of what your muscles feel like when tense (if you're tense all the time this may not be obvious to you) and, conversely, what they feel like when relaxed. By relaxing each muscle group from a point of tension, a greater degree of release of tension is possible. Many of our patients learn the skill in a few weeks, then become proficient at quickly scanning their bodies for signs of tension and quickly let it go as they go about their regular business. They can induce the same release of tension when in bed. Once our patients are able to utilize these techniques well, they needn't practice daily, but can return to the exercises occasionally. CD's and cassettes of these procedures are widely available. There are many different types of relaxation techniques. We encourage our patients to find a method that suits them and then persist with it.

## Eating, Drinking and Smoking

Many tinnitus patients receive advice to abstain from alcohol, caffeine, cheese, chocolate and a host of other things. There's little or no evidence to support most of this advice. There's some evidence that alcohol can make tinnitus temporarily more intrusive for some people. It is clear from that evidence, however, that for many more people alcohol either makes no difference <u>or it helps</u> because it makes them more relaxed. A special diet is sometimes suggested in the management of some ear disorders (such as a low sodium diet for *endolymphatic hydrops*), but for most people, restrictions in diet are unlikely to lead to less intrusive tinnitus but will simply make life miserable. Having said that, there's some sense in paying attention to diet when trying to achieve better sleep. Most of us are aware of the sedative effects of alcohol and it can sometimes help in falling to sleep. However, it can cause more disturbed sleep, particularly later in the night and of course reliance on alcohol to solve problems brings with it risks of other serous health-related problems. Caffeine and nicotine are stimulants and won't help you get to sleep either. Many people who wake in the night have tea or coffee because that's what they do in the daytime to "relax." At night their stimulating properties often become more apparent and our advice is to avoid these substances for a few hours before bedtime and entirely during the night.

If we're hungry we may have difficulty sleeping. Equally, if we have just had a large meal before bedtime, we may struggle to fall asleep. As with most things, it's about finding an appropriate balance and incorporating this into a routine that suits your lifestyle and usual bedtime. We advise our patients not to eat in the middle of the night.

### Bathing and Exercise

A bath can be relaxing before bed but it also brings about a change in body temperature so it's advisable to have a bath some time before bed to allow your body temperature to return to normal before retiring. Similarly, some exercise can help us to wind down provided that it's not too strenuous and done an hour or two before bed.

### Bedroom Activities

The bedroom needs to be a place where you can relax and feel calm. Therefore, it's important to restrict activities in this room to those that are consistent with resting and sleeping. This is why watching television in bed is generally not helpful. There are of course many people who find they can watch television in bed and still sleep well. Whilst this may be the case for some of us, it's not recommended as good practice and is definitely not a helpful strategy if your sleep is fragile in any way. Remember the makers of TV programs and commercials do not design them to send you to sleep.

### Clock Watching

It's very tempting to quickly check out the time when we're lying awake in the night. "How much longer do I have to lie here?" or "How much time have I got left to get some sleep?" Looking at the clock usually increases worry about sleep. If you need an alarm, face the clock away from the bed, otherwise you may try banishing it from the bedroom altogether.

## Reducing Time in Bed

People with concerns about their sleep will often spend a lot of time in bed in an effort to get more sleep. They think that if they lie there long enough that will make up for not having slept well. The time spent awake in bed in this way is a time of worry and fretting about sleep, emotions are high and associated thoughts are often unhelpful. Far from being restful or restorative, such time is often exhausting and leads to an association between bed and being awake and feeling tense. We encourage our patients to break this association by reducing the amount of time they spend in bed awake. There are four steps to doing this:

1. Go to bed when you feel tired rather than having a set bedtime.
2. If you're not asleep within 20-30 minutes after turning out the light, then get out of bed and go to a different room and do something restful and calming until you feel tired.
3. Go back to bed when you feel sleepy. If after another 20-30 minutes you're not asleep, return to Step 2 until you're again sleepy.
4. Get out of bed at the same time each day (even on weekends). This anchors your sleeping pattern at one end and provides you with a good base from which to develop a routine in your sleep.

We recognize that this can be difficult to do especially in the winter but it's known to be a powerful and effective means of regulating the sleep-wake cycle and breaking the frustrating and seemingly endless cycle of going to bed and tossing and turning all night.

## Daytime Napping

Sleeping during the day can disturb the sleep-wake cycle so we discourage this. Daytime napping can also undermine your confidence in coping with your sleeping pattern and may make you more anxious about your sleep. This can happen because you may conclude that you got through the day after a poor sleep the night before only because of that extra sleep you got in the afternoon. If you feel tired in the day, try to do something that increases your alertness such as some gentle exercise. By not sleeping in the day you minimize further disturbance to your sleep-wake cycle and you may discover that brief periods of sleepiness, such as most people experience after lunch, will pass.

## Worry Time

Our patients tell us that the most common problem keeping them awake is a busy mind. Bedtime is often the first time that a person has to think about things without other distractions. Often they are not just thinking about their tinnitus, but about everything that concerns them in their lives. Endlessly revising our various concerns at two in the morning seems to bring on particularly intense feelings of hopelessness or of impending catastrophe that is absent in the daytime when we're able to be more rational about issues. Usually, this worrying is not productive such as when you are actively working out how to solve a problem, but fruitless worrying where we go round and round in circles getting nowhere. Sometimes it can be helpful to schedule some worry-time, possibly in the early evening. Devote this time, maybe 20 minutes or so, to writing down the key issues concerning you and making some brief notes about what you might do about them. It may be that you record that you can do nothing about that problem for now. Some of our patients tell us that this allows them to switch off from worries when in bed by acknowledging to themselves that they have already done as much about that issue as they can for now and defer any further thinking until the next day.

## Imagery

Some people find it helpful to imagine a pleasant scene. This can be either entirely imaginary or taken from a fond memory or recent holiday. Imagining such a scene can reduce or eliminate a person's focus on a worrying idea. This seems to work better than deliberately trying not to think about something because we are all peculiarly bad at not thinking a thought. It we told you not to think about a pink elephant we would expect most of you to start thinking about an oversized garishly hued pachyderm. Another useful technique is *articulatory suppression.* In this technique you repeat a monosyllabic emotionally neutral word (such as 'the') in a quiet or silent voice to yourself. Many of our patients report that this helps to reduce focus on the thoughts and can also reduce focus on tinnitus. We suggest you combine a scheduled worry time as described above earlier in the evening with using articulatory suppression when in bed. Knowing that you have done all the useful things you can about a problem before going to bed minimizes the likelihood that it'll trouble you excessively when trying to sleep.

### Noise Enrichment

People naturally turn to external sources of sound such as radios and television to mask their tinnitus when in bed. Radios can, just as with television, stimulate and arouse us and we suggest that patients consider using commercially available sound generators that can sit on the bedside table if you believe that some sound is required. Radios can be used effectively by tuning to a station that is non-stimulating or by tuning it off the station so that a form of *white noise* can be heard. Ideally, if you use noise enrichment at bedtime, try to have the noise present in the room at a low level 24 hours a day so that it becomes an integral part of the bedroom environment rather than allowing it to become part of a dreadful bedtime ritual. Whenever any form of noise enrichment such as radios or sound generators are used, they should not be used at a level that masks or blocks out the tinnitus. Using sound to drown out tinnitus prevents you from developing a natural tolerance for the tinnitus (known as *habituation*) that occurs when we're exposed to a stimulus such as tinnitus over a sustained period of time.

## Should I Take Medication to Sleep?

NICE (National Institute for Clinical Excellence, www.nice.org.uk) is an independent UK organization responsible for providing national guidance on promoting good health and preventing and treating ill health. They've published guidance on the treatment of insomnia (Nice, 2004). In this section, we have very briefly summarized their main conclusions about the pharmacological treatment of insomnia.

Benzodiazepines (the type of drugs your doctor may have prescribed to help you sleep) and the newer sleeping pills (zaleplon, zolpidem and zopiclone: the so-called Z-drugs) are known as *hypnotics.* Generally, they should only be used for short periods of time and when used in this way can be very helpful in promoting sleep. Unfortunately, we develop tolerance for these drugs if we use them for longer periods (that is, they stop working as well or working at all) and we can become psychologically dependent upon them. That means that we can come to rely on them, even if they're not working well, and experience more sleep problems when we stop taking them. Many people develop some withdrawal symptoms (sometimes including tinnitus) when they stop using benzodiazepines. Long-term use of sleeping medication can actually make sleep problems worse and these drugs don't treat the underlying causes of your sleep problem. Psychological techniques such as cognitive behavioral therapy are a much more effective way of bringing about a real improvement in your sleep.

## How Can a Psychologist Help?

We all know that change can be difficult. Many of our patients have been successful in changing their sleeping patterns and other reactions to tinnitus by going through the processes outlined above; some have done it alone and some have done it with the support of a therapist. There's nothing wrong with asking for help. No one is able to do everything 100% independently. Many people ask for help from a mechanic when their car breaks down. So why should we be expected to deal with all problems in our lives without support?

Our emotions, thoughts and beliefs are invisible so it can be difficult to know how we are at times. Talking our problems through with a psychologist, who is experienced in understanding and identifying these aspects of how you are, just as a doctor knows how to identify what is wrong with you physically, can help you to understand more clearly how you're feeling and coping. They may also help you see what to do to resolve your problems. The techniques we've described in this chapter are drawn mostly from cognitive behavioral therapy. For help in finding a cognitive behavior therapist in your area consult the American Association for Behavioral and Cognitive Therapies (www.aabt.org) or the British Association of Behavioral and Cognitive Psychotherapists (www.babcp.com).

## Final Words

A significant factor in sleeping well is developing good sleeping habits. Whilst it might seem obvious that having tinnitus (it is a noise after all) will interfere with sleep, most of our patients are not troubled by their tinnitus at night. It's been found that people with insomnia often have other concerns or problems that are causing their sleep problems and addressing those concerns usually brings about some improvement. So it is with many of our tinnitus patients, where we have found that tinnitus may be exacerbating a long-term sleep problem or contributing to other worries that are themselves significantly affecting the quality of sleep. We hope that the contents of this chapter have given you some ideas for improving your sleep and we wish you a very goodnight.

## References

American Psychiatric Association (2000). <u>Diagnostic Criteria From DSM-IV-TR</u> (2000). Washington DC: American Psychiatric Association.

NICE. (2004). Guidance on the use of zaleplon, zolpidem and zopiclone for the short-term management of insomnia. Technology Appraisal 77.

## Additional Reading

We have given a brief outline of the nature of sleep and the effects of sleep loss. Take care when searching online for further information. The Internet contains some very useful material on sleep but also much that is misleading, frightening, and just plain wrong. Books can be a good source of information, but again, the purported facts or claims may be inaccurate or not scientifically based. More information about the perspective that we have offered can be found in the following books:

<u>Sleepfaring: A Journey through the Science of Sleep</u> by Professor Jim Horne of Loughborough University's Sleep Research Unit in the UK (Oxford University Press: NY, 2006) and <u>The Psychological Treatment of Insomnia</u> by Professor Colin Espie, Director of the Sleep Research Laboratory at the University of Glasgow, (Wiley:

Chichester, 1991). Also by Colin Espie, <u>Overcoming Insomnia and Sleep Problems: A Self-Help Guide Using Cognitive Behavioral Techniques</u> (Constable & Robinson Ltd., London, 2006).

# CHAPTER NINE

# Concentration

## Gerhard Andersson, PhD

*Linköping University and Karolinska Institutet, Sweden*

## Laurence McKenna, PhD

*Royal National Throat, Nose & Ear Hospital, London*

---

**Dr. Andersson** is professor of clinical psychology at Linköping University, Sweden. He is also guest professor at the Karolinska Institutet, Sweden. Apart from his research he also spends his time as a clinician working with tinnitus patients. Professor Andersson has done research and published papers on various aspects of tinnitus, including cognitive behavioral therapy, cognitive processes, brain imaging and personality. He is also the author of three books about tinnitus. Professor Andersson often lectures about tinnitus and advocates a multidisciplinary approach to its treatment. Probably his most important contribution to the field is development of Internet-delivered treatment of tinnitus distress.

**Dr. McKenna** has worked as a clinical psychologist at the Royal National Throat Nose & Ear Hospital for the past 24 years. During this time he has been involved in the study of tinnitus and other audiological disorders and in the psychological management of patients with these problems. He is head of the team of psychologists working in Adult Audiological Medicine and is a member of the cochlear implant team. Other work at Guy's and St Thomas' Hospitals in London has included the assessment and management of patients with neurological disorders, medico-legal work, management of attempted suicide patients, cochlear implantation and sleep disorders. He is an honorary lecturer at the Ear Institute (UCL) and Visiting Fellow at the University of Bristol.

---

## Introduction

In this chapter we'll provide a description of concentration problems common among people with problematic tinnitus. We'll also give a brief review of the current state of knowledge regarding tinnitus and concentration. Finally, we'll provide a few suggestions for dealing with concentration problems.

## What do we Mean by Concentration Problems?

When we see a tinnitus patient we always ask if tinnitus disrupts the ability to concentrate and focus on what is relevant in life. This is motivated by the fact that a majority of people in our tinnitus clinics report that their concentration is affected by their tinnitus. While disrupted concentration might not be the first thing that springs to mind if you're asked about your tinnitus, you're likely to agree when we ask you directly if you ever feel that you find it hard to stay focused all day long and concentrate when your tinnitus is bad. In fact, when tinnitus patients in a research study by Tyler and Baker (1983) were asked to list the problems they had with their tinnitus, the third most common response was concentration difficulties. In our own studies, we've asked directly in an interview, "Does tinnitus affect your concentration?" As many as 70% said that it did.

It's important to be clear that all people sometimes find it hard to concentrate. When we write about concentration problems here we mean occasions when you feel that your tinnitus negatively influences your ability to manage everyday activities such as reading, listening, remembering, planning, and other activities that require that you can concentrate. You might recognize this problem but not attribute it to your tinnitus. We'll get back to that, but please note that tinnitus is just one of many causes of concentration problems. In fact, it can also be the other way around. For quite a few patients we've seen it's when they concentrate on something that they're interested in that they experience their tinnitus as less apparent and annoying.

In order to be able to understand concentration problems we need to introduce three concepts that are well known in cognitive psychology. They will help us to further understand the different ways concentration and cognitive abilities might fail. The concepts will also be helpful when we present advice on how you can improve your concentration.

The first thing we think of is encoding. Basically, this has to do with how we take in information from our senses. If we take vision for instance, we need to have light, and have the object we look at an appropriate distance (not too far away). Moreover, we're helped if we know what we're looking at. For example, we can more easily encode an object we're familiar with than something unknown (like for instance an animal we've never seen before or never heard about). Encoding is of course crucial for the other senses as well, such as hearing. We need to be able to hear, or "take in," otherwise our brain has very little to rely on later in the process.

Our brain is usually extremely clever and often manages to "fill in the gaps" when pieces of information are missing in the process, but then we have already moved to the second step namely *elaboration*. At this stage the information is processed and links are made with other memories of names, places, time and various aspects that will ensure that the information is located in the right place in memory. Sometimes this can be a very quick process, such as when we recognize something as very familiar. At other times it can be harder. When we know little about the topic, or if we're distracted in various ways, elaboration becomes more difficult.

The third concept is *retrieval*. This is where the information is "retrieved" from memory or when we make use of stored information in the brain. We can distinguish between active and passive retrieval. For example, if we were to ask you to recall as many cities as you can remember in Europe, the number would probably be impressive, but not huge. If instead we give you a list of hundreds of cities in Europe and ask you to say if you recognize them or not, this would require less effort and you'd probably "recognize" far more cities than the ones you could remember during "free recall." Actually, the same applies when it comes to everyday activities. You'll probably not remember in great detail all your activities two days ago. But if we had monitored your activities with a video camera, you would recognize all of the content in the resulting film and be very surprised if we added something you felt you had not experienced (like, for instance, if we edit the film and add a gorilla in your living room). We elaborate on these issues since we know that tinnitus patients often judge themselves from how well they feel they perform when "trying to remember" and not from their ability to recognize. This process is described in Figure 9-1 below.

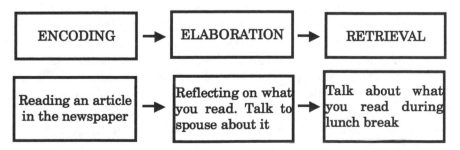

Figure 9-1: Encoding, elaboration and retrieval process

### What are the Effects of your Tinnitus on Concentration?

In this section we'll focus on the ways tinnitus might interfere with concentration. The literature on this topic is rather limited, but as we've already mentioned it's common to report concentration problems in association with tinnitus. What kind of problems do patients report? For some, tinnitus makes it more difficult to focus on conversations. A patient might say, "I can't focus on what people say and only hear my tinnitus. I give up after a while." Another common problem can be that it's in silence, and when the person is trying to read a book or just watching television after a long day at work, it can be reflected as: "I don't notice my tinnitus so much during the day. It's when I get home and sit down in front of television that it becomes its worst. I can't concentrate or focus on anything but the tinnitus. Reading is impossible. I usually put on some music instead."

Concentration problems can differ. Some report that their mind "wanders" and that they start thinking about other things than, for example, the newspaper they're reading. This happens to all of us, but for a person with tinnitus it can be the tinnitus sound(s) that attracts the attention. Various thoughts and reactions can occur. It might even be that you "monitor" your tinnitus to check if it's louder, different or in any way changing. Then again, the distraction can be to just anything, but you attribute your concentration problems to tinnitus, even when there are other things that distract you. For example, problems at work, lack of money, or family problems can impinge on ability to focus and concentrate. Another way to lose concentration temporarily is when you "go blank." This again might happen to all of us, but is known to occur when you're depressed. Then instead of the mind wandering off to other things than the task at hand, it just goes blank. For you who have problems with sleep this might sound familiar. Being very tired increases the risk of going blank, and when your mind goes blank tinnitus might still be very much present although you might not particularly focus on it.

In order to continue the discussion here we need to introduce the concept of *working memory.* It's now widely agreed by most psychologists that human memory consists of different components that act separately and together to help us filter and remember information. For example, we distinguish between *short-term memory* and *long-term memory.* Short-term memory is usually called "working memory." This is the memory system that holds the input while interpretation of it is worked out. For example, in order to be able to read a long sentence, you'll need to have the first part or words of the sentence in your working memory to be able to put the latter parts in context and understand the whole sentence. Another example is when you're given a telephone number and leave the phone to find a piece of paper to write it down. You need to remember the number just long enough in your working memory so that you can write it down. Then it can disappear (otherwise you wouldn't need to write it down). Working memory can be disrupted and we have reasons to believe that tinnitus in some circumstances can disrupt working memory, leading to concentration and memory problems. In fact, those minor "disruptions" might be a reason why tinnitus attracts attention. For example, you might recognize that you notice your tinnitus when it interferes with something you want to focus on, like listening to what is being said during a meeting at work. However, from a research point of view, it's not always easy to confirm the experiences of our patients in the laboratory. In fact, when we test our patients in experiments using established tests of cognitive function (for example, a test in which the task is to replace numbers with symbols), we sometimes find that they might perform pretty well on these more "objective" tests, while still having problems with concentration in their daily life.

Perhaps one reason is that all attention is focused in the test situation in the laboratory while in other settings tinnitus "wins" and grabs more attention. As we'll return to later in this chapter, hearing loss might also play a major role in this process. One of us did two studies on the neuropsychological functioning in tinnitus patients. As might be suspected, there was clear evidence of more self-reported problems, but when hearing impaired people without tinnitus were used as controls, few differences on objective measures were found.

In other words, we cannot distinguish if it is tinnitus or hearing impairment that is causing the problems. Please note that we are not saying the last word here since there is conflicting evidence. For example, many researchers have suggested that attending to tinnitus is indeed an important factor. We know that some people rarely notice or attend to their tinnitus (this is in fact very common), whereas other people might find it harder not to listen to their tinnitus and cannot escape its intrusive character. Fortunately, this rarely happens 24 hours a day. You may very well recognize this. Sometimes you notice your tinnitus more and sometimes less. The loudness of your tinnitus is of course one factor, but it doesn't tell the full story.

You might notice your tinnitus <u>even when it's not louder than usual</u>. For some of the patients we've met, it's factors other than the loudness that make them focus more on their tinnitus. One way attention to tinnitus has been studied is to see how fast patients respond to sounds (for example, reaction time). Briefly, this research has found that at least some tinnitus patients listen selectively to tinnitus-like sounds. In one experiment conducted by Hallam and coworkers (2004), they found evidence suggesting that the cognitive problems among tinnitus patients were related to <u>the ability to control attention</u>, in particular when they asked their study participants to do two things simultaneously.

This leads us over to another possibility. It could be that tinnitus and sounds in the environment interact and that this has an influence on concentration. One of us tested this notion in a study (Andersson et al., 2002) in which 20 tinnitus subjects and 20 control subjects without tinnitus were asked to do a cognitive test. This was the digit-symbol test, actually the one we referred to previously in which the test person is asked to replace symbols for numbers by using a "key." (For instance the symbol ¤ would stand for number 2, and so forth). They completed the test in three auditory conditions: silence, masking, and intermittent masking (broadband noise that was set to totally mask the tinnitus). The hypothesis was that tinnitus would be most distractive in silence (when it's heard most clearly).

First, results showed marked overall differences between tinnitus subjects and control subjects on all three conditions. The tinnitus patients had lower scores on the test (that is, they were less able to substitute symbols from the number key). The second main finding was that the patients had lower scores on the digit-symbol test during the intermittent masking condition compared with the masking condition. The implications of this is that sounds that come and go might lead to concentration problems as the tinnitus is masked temporarily and then returns after a short break when it's no longer masked. This can make tinnitus more noticeable than if it had been around constantly (that is, audible). The effects of tinnitus on long-term memory are not well known. However, long-term memory can be sensitive to bias—in other words, a tendency to selectively remember certain things more clearly and other things less clearly. This has been studied by one of us in a study on *autobiographical memory* in tinnitus patients (Andersson et al., 2003), which was inspired by research done with depressed patients. In depression research, a consistent observation has been that depressed patients have difficulties generating specific autobiographical memories (meaning from a specific time and place, e.g., "the day I lost my keys when cycling"). Usually, this is tested by providing subjects with a cue-word (for example, "happy"), and giving them 1 minute to generate a specific memory. Using such a test in one study it was found that compared to control participants, tinnitus patients had some difficulty retrieving specific memories.

Another type of bias has to do with selective attention. This might also be relevant for our understanding of tinnitus. For example, patients with anxiety disorder selectively attend to information related to their concern (for example, shapes that remind a snake phobic of a snake). We call this type of selective attention *cognitive bias.* While this has been investigated in chronic pain, there has been relatively little research on tinnitus. One of us has studied this aspect of tinnitus in a series of studies. So far, we have only indications that tinnitus patients selectively attend to information related to tinnitus (for example, words reminding them of their tinnitus).

In summary, the available evidence suggests that tinnitus patients show some signs of cognitive bias, but it's unclear whether patients think in an anxious (selective attention) or depressive (memory bias) manner, or both. It could possibly be the case that subgroups of tinnitus patients exist in terms of their cognitive bias. That is, it could be that two forms of distressed tinnitus patients exist, one being characterized by depressive symptoms and the other by anxiety symptoms.

## The link between Concentration Problems and Annoyance

There are many reasons why tinnitus becomes annoying. If you follow the research literature on tinnitus you'll find many references to emotional well-being. Often the researchers mean symptoms such as depression and anxiety and how they can make the experience of tinnitus even worse. However, we think that concentration problems are sometimes forgotten as an explanation of why you might feel annoyed by your tinnitus. In fact, if we investigate this possibility in our data, we find a relatively strong association between the extent to which tinnitus patients report "cognitive failures" and how disturbed they are by their tinnitus. You might wonder what kind of cognitive failures people report? This has not been investigated in any detail, but in our clinical practices we've seen many forms of concentration problems among our patients. These include, for example, problems with reading long texts, difficulties following conversations (in particular, for longer periods), memory lapses, and difficulties engaging in recreational activities where there's a demand on concentration (for example, remembering turns when dancing). For some, it might be the case that tinnitus is so irritating that it becomes hard to focus on anything else. Degree of hearing loss is always important to consider since hearing impairment can result in the very same problems. We will turn to this issue next.

### Is it Just Tinnitus?

We can't get past this issue since it's often not <u>only</u> tinnitus that is responsible for concentration problems. We've hinted at this possibility earlier in the chapter, but now we'll focus on these other plausible reasons.

We begin with hearing loss. Most people with tinnitus have hearing loss as well. For many this is as problematic as the tinnitus, but for other reasons. Hearing loss can be a communication handicap, and can be highly visible in social settings. Communication breakdown can occur and misunderstandings are frequent. While hearing aids help, they're not a "cure" and residual problems often persist in noisy environments. Finding it hard to concentrate and maintain a conversation is a challenge for many individuals with impaired hearing. Do you recognize this from your life? Even mild hearing loss can lead to concentration problems and fatigue, which is another common reason why concentration might fail. For some people we see in our clinics it can be hard to differentiate what problems are caused by tinnitus and what problems should be attributed to hearing loss. In fact, it can be that both problems interact (meaning that one plus one is more than two). For example, straining to hear might make you tired and you tend to focus on your tinnitus instead (which requires no effort since it's always there in the background).

The long-term consequences of hearing loss can also be that you get used to not being able to hear and "give up." We know that listening requires some "guessing" and filling in the gaps, and this is something that all people do in conversations. By the way, this is a reason why it can be more difficult for you to communicate in a noisy setting when you listen in a language or to a strong accent you're not so familiar with—you don't have the same possibilities to fill in the gaps as when you listen in your native language. When hearing has been impaired for a long time you might lose some of your abilities to guess and to fill in the gaps. Researchers have referred to this as your *internal dialogue.* This is somewhat compromised by hearing loss. In any case, when we talk about concentration problems with our tinnitus patients we need to be careful as some problems might be the result of hearing loss and hence require solutions that incorporate ways to improve the listening and communication situation as well.

Another factor that can have adverse effects on your concentration abilities is psychological distress. We know from research that many people with severe tinnitus are depressed and anxious and some of these problems can be of such an extent that you might fulfill the criteria for a psychiatric diagnosis of major depression and/or an anxiety disorder. This aspect is commented on elsewhere in this book (see Chapter 4), but we bring it up here since it can have consequences for your concentration abilities. For example, if you're feeling depressed, you're likely to have concentration and memory problems. If you're anxious it might be that your attention is drawn toward things you fear or worry about, which might well include fears about your tinnitus becoming worse and other aspects of your health.

A third aspect relates to the effects of medication and possibly other health conditions. For example, diabetes can be associated with impaired concentration. Some of the commonly prescribed medications can have fatigue and concentration problems as side effects. While not necessarily related to a health condition, aging can result in concentration problems. There are of course also cases in which an undetected brain dysfunction can be behind the concentration problems.

### Specific Advice for Improving your Concentration

There are several research studies showing that you can benefit from training your concentration skills. Here we'll present a few exercises we use in tinnitus treatment (Kaldo & Andersson, 2004).

The first thing to do is select activities in which you feel your concentration is disrupted by your tinnitus. You should pick at least one. Here are a few examples:

- reading (newspapers, journals, Web pages, leaflets);
- listening (lectures, dinner table, radio or TV);
- planning or being creative (plan for vacation, a work asignment, come up with new ideas);
- study or learn something new (a language, new knowledge, memorize, poems, stories);
- control (spotting errors, sort out economy);
- solving problems (everyday problems, crosswords, games);
- write (shorter or longer texts, diaries, letters, emails);
- try your own idea.

Once you've done this, we have a list of recommendations that you can consider when tackling your problems. The first 6 of the following 12 ideas deal with arranging for you to <u>take pauses</u>.

**1. Pause your ongoing activities for a restricted period of time, preferably 15-30 minutes. Do not work longer than 45 minutes on a task.**

<u>Comments</u>: Write down and plan when the pauses will occur. It might be easier for you if you plan in advance. If you say to yourself "I just need to do one more thing…" things easily get out of hands. Why not consider using an alarm clock or program your computer or cellular phone when a break is due? Please note that the time required to do a certain task might vary between tasks and their location/setting. It might for example not be possible to leave a meeting after 45 minutes however much you would like to do so. It's also of course depending on the effort required from you. For some tasks your concentration abilities might last much less than 45 minutes. If you know that in advance, you can plan pauses ahead of exhaustion. When you start, it might be a good idea to have a few extra pauses and then reduce them when you notice that it works.

**2. Decide in advance the amount of work you should complete before you have your break. Even if you have not finished, you will still need to take your pause after 45 minutes.**

<u>Comments</u>: This is an alternative to letting the clock decide when it's time to have a break. Divide the work into smaller parts and decide how much work you should put in before a break. However, if

you reach the limit of 45 minutes it might be a good idea to have a break anyway. This can be important as your brain might need some rest and recovery after the hard work. You may feel frustrated when pausing from an ongoing activity. One way to deal with this is to write down a few key words to remind you where you were before the break.

### 3. Ask someone to remind you to take a break.

Comments: It might be easier to have a break if you have it together with someone. It can also provide you with an opportunity for conversation. Even if you decide to have the break on your own, you can still ask someone (for example, a colleague or family member) to remind you about the break.

### 4. Do something nice during the break as a reward for the work you have done.

Comments: While this may seem obvious, we often forget to reward ourselves for the work we've done and instead we rush to the next assignment or task. There are many ways you can give yourself small rewards such as a nice walk, a drink, or some fruit, just to give a few examples. For many of us, social contact is also rewarding and a telephone call to a close friend or partner can also be a reward. Obviously, some of the things we would like to use to reward ourselves are not healthy (for example, a cigarette) and should therefore not be used.

### 5. Use relaxation, positive imagery and physical activity.

Comments: Many of us work in office settings and it can be good for our concentration over the day to relax by taking a brief pause using just a deep breath or imagining something positive like a beach or a winter landscape. Also, if you sit most of the day, exercise in particular is often beneficial. Remember that small exercises like taking the stairs instead of the elevator can also be beneficial and have a relaxing effect. Using inner images is also a very useful and commonly practiced way to enhance memory. For instance, if you mentally "rehearse" the day you have in front of you, this "practice" can enhance your ability to remember the things you need to do.

## 6. Use your pause in activities to think things over.

Comments: One way to improve concentration can be to revisit the situation in your thoughts. You can think about the situation without actually working on a solution. For example, if you read something, you should put away the book while you think about what you just read. If you work in front of a computer, stay away from it (for example, don't have your break in front of the computer checking the news on the Web or your incoming e-mails).

A second category of advice has to do with planning, structuring and prioritizing. Planning can alleviate and prevent stress. If you know in advance what to expect during a day it can be easier to stay concentrated. If you, on the other hand, are overloaded with work, your chances to keep concentration will decrease. You might need to find a balance between how much you want to do and how much you can reasonably do within the limits of your resources. You might argue that you didn't need to plan before you got your tinnitus. However, planning can result in better work whether we have tinnitus or not.

## 7. Divide a task into smaller steps. Count each step as a task on its own.

Comments: This can be a very helpful way to boost your confidence and prevent a sense of failure. You might also discover that certain parts of the task can be skipped, reduced, done later or delegated to someone else. Each step can differ in length (in terms of time), but should not exceed the limits we discussed above regarding when it's time to have a break (for example, not more than 45 minutes). You can benefit from making each step clearly defined. If you have the task of learning some material, for example, you might divide the process up into several steps. If you read one chapter in a book, you might write a brief summary of it. If you're planning to paint the house, this would definitely be a complex task. This could perhaps be divided into discussing with friends and neighbors if they can assist; decide what color to use; buy paint; clean the brushes. These are but a few examples of smaller but still relevant steps. This advice fits in very well with the other suggestions we gave regarding breaks, writing down and crossing out what you have achieved, and last but not least, give yourself a reward for each step.

## 8. Write down a list and cross out each thing you have done.

Comments: We know from experience that some of our tinnitus patients (in common with depressed persons) ignore or forget their progress and only see the mistakes they've made. Writing a diary or making a list of things you plan and then using the same list to document what you've done can be an intrinsically rewarding experience. Maybe you might already do this sometimes. This can serve both as an aid for memory and as a way to give yourself feedback. Don't criticize yourself too much. A small step can be important, and a partly completed step can often be supplemented with an additional task to finally be completed.

## 9. Start with an easier task and gradually continue with more advanced tasks.

Comments: It can be even more important if you have stayed away from concentration-demanding tasks for awhile. It's perfectly understandable that you'll not immediately function on the same level as you did before. Also remember that it's indeed common to get tired when you're dealing with either complicated or boring tasks. This is not something that concerns only people with tinnitus. Many other problems, including hearing loss, can contribute to the concentration problems as much, or even more than, the tinnitus. We recommend that you not start with the difficult goals. By starting with an easier task you increase the likelihood of success.

## 10. Prioritize and do not take on too many assignments.

Comments: Wanting to do something is not the same as getting it done. Various strategies exist for someone who needs to set up boundaries. All people, regardless of whether they have tinnitus or not, need to find a balance between their resources and their limits. Stress can impede your ability to function in a focused manner. You may need to practice how to say "No" to some invitations, and this can be trickier than it seems. In particular, if you fear failure and are sensitive to being rejected, it might become even more problematic for you to turn down requests. But in the long-run this can be the only way to handle the situation and prevent being exhausted.

**11. Make it easier for yourself. For example, use your diary, notes, arrange the setting so that you will be reminded, ask other people to remind you, and use your cellular phone, calendar or e-mail for reminders.**

<u>Comments</u>: You can gain a lot of time by not having too many thoughts in your head at the same time. If you're relieved from the pressure to remember, it will become easier to stay focused on the task at hand. To write things down is one obvious way you might already practice. However, you might need some additional assistance by arranging your environment so that it becomes easier to remember things. For example, by rehearsing for yourself what is due to occur during the next day, you can become better prepared. Perhaps you can put the needed papers in your bag before you leave work. The dinner party you plan may be planned together with someone close to you. You might be helped by notes placed at strategic positions, or why not electronic reminders from your computer or cellular phone? Reminders that have a date associated with them should be put in your calendar. You could also email yourself a reminder.

**12. Focus on one thing at a time.**

<u>Comments</u>: This is something to strive for, since being more focused makes you more effective in the long-run. Obviously, when you're stuck, it might be better to do something else, but there's a risk if you give up too quickly or if you jump from one task to the other. Remember also that it often takes harder work to change paths constantly than to do what you do in a balanced and focused manner.

### A Few More Words

There are several other ways you can influence your concentration. It's often possible to influence your surroundings, like light and heating conditions. Your mood and alertness can be influenced by your eating habits. Your tinnitus can at least be partially handled by introducing competing sounds, a form of "sound enrichment." If you feel very irritated and annoyed by tinnitus it can be worth considering the role of acceptance (see Chapter 6). Not in the sense of liking your tinnitus, but rather acceptance of the facts of life and the willingness to move on and focus on the things you want to do in your life. For some, this can mean that you deliberately challenge yourself. For instance, if you're very disturbed by background sounds, it can be a good idea to practice to act and live with background sounds in your environment.

We all know that tinnitus can be a difficult challenge for the sufferer. But we also know that many people manage and even do quite well in spite of tinnitus by devoting some time to find strategies to manage concentration problems. Your tinnitus problem can be decreased since concentration problems are among the most commonly reported problems among tinnitus sufferers. By being strategic and focused, you have a good chance of improving your memory and concentration skills.

## References

Andersson, G., Khakpoor, A., & Lyttkens, L. (2002). Masking of tinnitus and mental activity. *Clinical Otolaryngology,* 27, 270-274.

Andersson, G., Ingerholt, C., & Jansson, M. (2003). Autobiographical memory in patients with tinnitus. *Psychology & Health,* 18, 667-675.

Hallam, R. S., McKenna, L., & Shurlock, L. (2004). Tinnitus impairs cognitive efficiency. *International Journal of Audiology,* 43, 218-226.

Kaldo, V., & Andersson, G. (2004). Kognitiv beteendeterapi vid tinnitus. [Cognitive-behavioural treatment of tinnitus]. Lund: Studentlitteratur.

Tyler, R. S., & Baker, L. J. (1983). Difficulties experienced by tinnitus sufferers. *Journal of Speech and Hearing Disorders,* 48, 150-154.

## Recommended Reading

Andersson, G., Baguley, D. M., McKenna, L., & McFerran, D. J. (2005). Tinnitus: A Multidisciplinary Approach. London: Whurr.

Andersson, G., & Kaldo, V. (2006). Cognitive-behavioral therapy with applied relaxation. In R. S. Tyler (Ed.), Tinnitus Treatment: Clinical Protocols (pp. 96-115). New York: Thieme.

Andersson, G., & McKenna, L. (2006). The role of cognition in tinnitus. *Acta Otolaryngologica,* 126, 39-43.

Baddeley, A. D. (1986). Working Memory. Oxford: Oxford University Press.

Henry, J., & Wilson, P. (2002). <u>Tinnitus. A Self-Management Guide for the Ringing in your Ears</u>. Boston: Allyn & Bacon.

# CHAPTER TEN

# Sound Therapy Options

## Grant D. Searchfield, PhD
*The University of Auckland*

---

**Dr. Searchfield** obtained his PhD in Audiology from The University of Auckland where he is currently a lecturer in Aural Rehabilitation. He is director of the University's Hearing and Tinnitus Clinic and undertakes tinnitus research from his laboratory at the School of Population Health. He has published research papers in diverse areas of tinnitus study including auditory physiology and sound therapy. Dr. Searchfield is a regular contributor to international conferences in tinnitus management, and is an international editorial associate for the Journal of the American Academy of Audiology.

---

"A horrid stillness first invades the ear,
and in that silence we the tempest fear."
J. Dryden

Almost everyone with tinnitus has the experience that their tinnitus is worse when they're in a quiet room, and most will also be aware of some sounds that make their tinnitus more difficult to hear. However, the interaction between an external sound and tinnitus is not a simple one. The complex relationship is because tinnitus exists even when no external sound is present, and it appears to be coded, at least in some ways, unlike external sounds. Tinnitus isn't caused by physical sound vibrations; instead it's the brain's picture of a sound. Tinnitus does not obey all the rules which normally apply to listening to an external sound (Tyler, 2000). For example, tinnitus may be difficult to *mask* (cover) even with very loud sounds close to the pitch of the tinnitus. The unusual way that sound interacts with tinnitus means that sound therapy isn't as simple as covering one sound with another.

Sounds can evoke a wide range of responses in a person, including emotional reactions, muscle contractions and change in heart rate. When sound is being used to defeat tinnitus, it's important that the positive effects of sound are being promoted and any negative effects are minimized. It serves little purpose to replace tinnitus with a more annoying sound. In this chapter I'll introduce some of the principles surrounding the use of sound to treat tinnitus and, in addition, various "sound" or "acoustic" therapies and the devices developed to implement these treatments.

## Attention and Distraction

"Learning to ignore things is one of the great paths to inner peace."
R.J. Sawyer

Sound is used in many tinnitus therapies to distract attention away from tinnitus and to reduce the brain's ability to fully process tinnitus activity. In our daily activities a mixture of sounds reaches our ears and the auditory system needs to choose the relevant sounds from the background noise. For normal hearing we must ignore irrelevant information so that we don't become distracted, but we must also be able to hear and react to important (potentially dangerous) events which we're not focusing on. For example, while crossing the street conversing with someone, we need to react to the sound of an ambulance siren. If we don't, we end up needing the ambulance (or worse)! It appears that the brain's attention is attracted to tinnitus as if it was an important sound. Have you ever noticed how you can hear your name above the background noise babble at a party? Tinnitus seems to have the same attention-capturing characteristics. The effect of tinnitus is partly dependent upon the attention given to it. A decrease in attention to tinnitus through distraction should lead to its reduction. This distraction can be achieved using tactics such as searching for and identifying sounds other than tinnitus. Henry and Wilson, two Australian psychologists, suggested some simple attention strategies can be applied easily for this purpose. They suggest that by exerting control over attention, tinnitus-related distress will be reduced. I suggest using their technique to alternate attention from tinnitus to others sounds:

"Focus your awareness on the noises in your head - tune into the noises. What can you hear?...Now quickly redirect your attention. Focus on external noises in the room and outside...notice you can only focus on one thing at a time." (Henry & Wilson, 2002, page 106)

Attention diversion attempts to move the sufferer's focus away from the tinnitus and onto some other object or action. At the same time imagery training can be used to evoke strong positive sensations associated with tinnitus such as imagining tinnitus as if it were rain, surf or a waterfall. An optimal level of sound that facilitates distraction of attention away from the tinnitus will be the most efficient level for controlling tinnitus.

## Masking

"I hear a sound so fine there's nothing lives 'Twixt it and silence."
                                                                J.S. Knowles

Masking is the process of covering, or partially covering, tinnitus with sound. Masking is one of the simplest (and oldest) methods for treating tinnitus. Medical historians attribute the 19th Century French physician Jean-Marie Itard (1775-1838) with development of masking. Itard suggested listening to sounds made by fires burning different wood types - burning damp wood would mask high frequency tinnitus due to hissing sounds while low frequency tinnitus could be masked by the roaring sound of dry-seasoned firewood. Hearing aids were the first electronic devices used to manage tinnitus. Saltzman and Ernor (1947) found that amplification of sounds by simple hearing aids was successful in "crowding out" tinnitus (Saltzman & Ersner, 1947). Clinically, practical masking was first systematically implemented by Jack Vernon, PhD, of Portland Oregon, in the mid-1970s when ear-level hearing aid-style electronic maskers became available commercially (see also Chapter 14).

Masking either causes tinnitus to become inaudible (complete masking) or, with lower masker levels, allows the tinnitus to be heard above the noise (partial masking). Masking tends to reduce the prominence or apparent loudness of the tinnitus. It's thought that masking causes the neural circuit processing tinnitus to be too busy with real sound to attend to it. Tinnitus masking is based on the observation that masking sounds and the tinnitus they cover should also be ignored. Benefit may be obtained from a masking device if the patient finds the noise more pleasant to listen to than their tinnitus, or if it helps them ignore their tinnitus. It can help if the masker sound is relaxing. Masking can have an additional advantage in that it's empowering; the person with tinnitus can determine when they will or will not hear their tinnitus.

The importance of the type of sound made by a masker is debated. The ability of a sound to mask tinnitus varies between patients and no single masking sound has been shown to be universally successful. Some researchers have concluded that the most effective maskers are those with broad bandwidths, containing a wide spectrum of sound, while other studies have shown more effective masking occurs when the masking sound is close in pitch to that of the tinnitus. Some patients find traditional masking sounds to be equally annoying as their tinnitus and cannot continue masking as a treatment option.

The inner ear is divided into bands of filters; if noise fills one of these bands it can swamp another sound in that band (see Chapter 7). Normally a sound has to be in the same band to be masked. In 34% of tinnitus cases studied by Feldmann (1971) the masking sound was most successful when the frequency content of the masking sound matched that of the tinnitus. In 32% of cases the masking sound had no similarity to the frequency spectrum of the tinnitus, and 11% of cases were unmaskable. Because the pitch of a tinnitus masking sound is not critical, it's believed that sounds interfere with tinnitus - not at the inner ear, but at the level of the brain. This also can explain why masking sounds in one ear can mask tinnitus in the other ear. This effect is known as "central masking" and occurs because the brain has difficulty separating signals containing similar information.

Masking can be achieved using hearing aids, ear-level tinnitus maskers or combination instruments and various types of sound-generating devices (for example, tabletop maskers, water fountains, radios, compact discs [CDs] and MP3/"ipod" devices). Variable success rates have been reported for the clinical use of tinnitus maskers. In a study by Schleuning, Johnson and Vernon (1980), 68% of participants who purchased maskers obtained partial relief and 15% obtained complete relief from their tinnitus, giving a combined success rate of 83%. However, other studies have shown less favorable results, with some studies indicating no significant difference in tinnitus relief between patients fitted with a masker and those who had counseling alone.

I think that masking is often an effective management option, especially when the person is seeking some degree of control. Masking allows sufferers to determine when they don't wish to hear their tinnitus. Masking is normally provided with some counseling. The basic counseling provided to patients generally includes information about the cause of tinnitus, the nature of their hearing loss, and the use of sound to provide relief from the annoyance of tinnitus.

Clinicians differ in their approach regarding setting the level of the masker noise relative to the tinnitus. Some advise complete masking of the tinnitus. This may not be possible for everybody. Other clinicians focus on (or try to achieve) a level where the tinnitus and masker are just about equal and both can be perceived (partial masking). Still other clinicians suggest that the masker be at the lowest level to provide relief, sometimes just audible (a lower level of partial masking). Research suggests that the less intense the masking sound, the more acceptable it is. In some cases the tinnitus may actually disappear for a period of time following a masker being turned off. This reduction is called *residual inhibition* or *post-masking* relief. If residual inhibition occurs it can last for as little as a few seconds to several days.

Some people with tinnitus attending my clinic ask, "Why would I want this masking sound, I already have enough noise in my head?" My answer is, "Well, silence would be great, but wouldn't you rather hear a sound you like and can control rather than the tinnitus?"

## Habituation

"At nine o'clock every morning the mill-wheel began to turn, and its roaring never stopped all day. For the first moments the noise was terrifying, was almost unbearable. Then, after a little, one grew accustomed to it. The thunder became, by reason of its very unintermittence, a perfect silence..."
A. Huxley

The human brain is capable of some interesting "tuning" capabilities. For example, if you have a sliver in your finger and aren't in a place where you can remove it right away, you sort of become accustomed to it. We call this *habituation*. Relative to hearing, if a sound is repeated over and over again and no danger results, we learn to ignore it. For example, if you're reading a book in your house while the wind blows outside and birds persistently chirp, within a short time most people will be "tuning out" these external sounds as they become engrossed in their reading. This process is called *auditory habituation*. It's just a decline in the tendency to respond to sounds that have become familiar due to repeated exposure. In our daily lives, this process allows us to ignore unimportant "background" sounds, yet respond appropriately to stimuli that are significant for our survival; for example, the sound of an ambulance siren that suddenly interrupts music in your car. A major benefit of auditory habituation is that it narrows down the range of sounds that grab our attention (Worden, 1976). The perception of tinnitus and its associated concentration problems may be the result of the brains inability to habituate, that is, to efficiently process and filter the signal creating tinnitus.

Hallam and colleagues proposed a habituation model of tinnitus perception (Hallam, Rachman, & Hinchcliffe, 1984). Their model suggests that tinnitus should normally be ignored but is not because the process of habituation is stopped. They suggest barriers to tinnitus habituation include: a relatively sudden change in input level (for example, a sudden hearing loss), persistent high levels of stress and anxiety (for example, a worsening of hearing loss), unnecessary worry (tinnitus equals brain tumor), or if the tinnitus fluctuates in quality (pitch) or intensity (loudness).

A high percentage of people with tinnitus are not severely bothered by it. Tinnitus annoyance sometimes decreases over time but may become more annoying in times of stress. Also, people who obtain the greatest success from tinnitus treatments often show high levels of positive self-beliefs and good coping strategies. The difference between a person who experiences tinnitus and one who "suffers" from it may be the person's ability to come to terms with tinnitus and habituate to it.

The goal of habituation therapy is to relegate tinnitus to being an unattended background sound. We don't hear all sounds in our daily environment because many aren't interesting or useful; for example, the hum of a computer fan, or sounds of wind blowing outdoors. The process of habituation involves reducing levels of tinnitus awareness to such a level that it doesn't receive attention. If there's no awareness of tinnitus, the tinnitus shouldn't be a problem. The first clinicians to use the concept of tinnitus habituation were psychologists. Subsequently several habituation-based approaches have developed which prescribe the use of hearing aids or sound generators (maskers).

The continuous presentation of sound by hearing aids or sound generators of any type might interfere with the neural code responsible for tinnitus (Chapter 3). Although there's no data to support this, many have suggested that long-term sound therapy might even result in permanent changes in the tinnitus code, perhaps even eliminating it.

There are different kinds of noise that can be used in sound therapy. Noise is characterized by spectrum, or the level of all its frequency components (see Chapter 7). Most maskers use a wide range of frequencies (called broadband), and some emphasize the low or high frequency regions. A broadband noise is usually recommended for sound therapies since it's assumed to be a "neutral" sound which creates a stable background noise somewhat similar to the random neural activity that's believed to be the neural code for silence. The ideal treatment sound would theoretically create mild stimulation of the entire population of neurons within the auditory pathways and be neutral so as not to negatively activate the attention and emotion centers of the brain.

There's little evidence to support the use of one therapeutic sound over another; some evidence suggests that more natural sounds are preferred to noise. In addition to hearing aids and sound generators, I also encourage people to listen to pleasant sounds whenever they're in quiet environments. Nature sounds, New Age relaxation music, and orchestral music are often excellent self-help sound therapy options. I recommend that sound is used at the lowest effective level that interacts with the tinnitus.

## Hearing Aids
"The empty vessel makes the greatest sound."
W. Shakespeare

Modern hearing aids are powerful tools for sound therapy (Searchfield, 2006). Hearing aids are used both for aiding communication and for providing a continuous means of sound enhancement. Often, tinnitus relief is the primary goal of hearing aids, especially if the hearing loss is only a minor concern. In the presence of hearing loss the fitting of hearing aids enables auditory input to return to more normal levels. Traditionally, hearing aids have been thought to help tinnitus by reducing the stress associated with straining to hear, by diverting attention away from tinnitus to other sounds and by partially masking or suppressing tinnitus by amplifying background sounds (Figure 10-1). Hearing aids can lead to less social isolation. That is, being involved in enjoyable social activities can divert attention from the tinnitus. Amplified speech sounds or music may result in greater demands on the brain's attention than noise. Also, the sounds amplified by hearing aids may interfere with the central auditory interpretation and processing of changed auditory activity that is responsible for tinnitus.

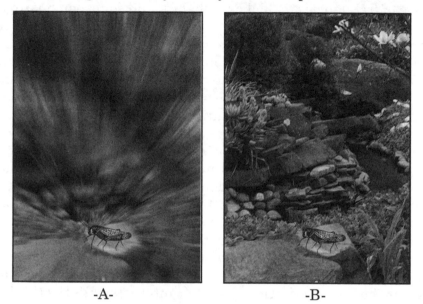

-A-                                    -B-

Figure 10-1: A simple visual representation of tinnitus and hearing loss

Imagine that the cricket represents a person's tinnitus and the background image represents background sounds. In "A" the person has a hearing loss, the background sound is indistinct and the cricket (tinnitus) is very clear.  In "B" the person has been fitted with a hearing aid, the background is clear and rich in detail and although the cricket (tinnitus) is still present it blends into the background and our attention is diverted to other features of the environment. The success of hearing aids in managing tinnitus often depends on how well background sounds can be made to blend with tinnitus.

There's accumulating evidence that changes occur in the organization of the hearing part of the brain following damage to the ear (see Chapter 3). Disruption of these sound processing regions of the brain has been suggested to result in tinnitus, much in the same way that loss of a limb can lead to reorganization of the brain and the "phantom" perception of pain. In some cases of *phantom limb* pain, stimulation of the area near the injury or use of artificial limbs has been shown to lead to a reduction in pain. Hearing aids may affect tinnitus in the same way. I encourage people with tinnitus to think of hearing aid use as physiotherapy for the ears - listening to sound around us to exercise the auditory portion of the brain.

When hearing aids are fitted just to help hearing, about 50% of wearers will notice benefit in reducing their tinnitus (Surr et al., 1985). If modern hearing aids are fitted with tinnitus as the prime concern, more people should find them successful. The use of hearing aids as a successful sound treatment for tinnitus is frequently dependent on the hearing aids being comfortable, avoiding loudness discomfort, and being tuned to allow maximum comfortable amplification of quiet sounds.

New "open fit" hearing aids have been shown to be very effective for this task. Open fit hearing aids are small appliances that hook over the ear with a slim "invisible" tube leading into the ear canal. They're designed especially for hearing losses in which hearing for low-pitched sounds is normal while a hearing loss exists for high-pitched sounds. The hearing loss is compensated for by amplification of sound within the frequency range of the hearing loss; good hearing areas are not affected. It's important that the hearing aids are used as much as possible throughout waking hours and care should be taken to prevent obstruction of natural sounds coming to the ear. Sometimes people with tinnitus localized in one ear, and hearing loss in both, ask me, "Why are you recommending two hearing aids?" The answer is that although tinnitus may be localized to one ear, it doesn't mean that the other ear cannot play a role in reducing it. Remember that tinnitus is a central representation of sound—not true sound. If you needed glasses would you settle for a monocle?

If patients have moderate hearing loss, combined hearing aids and noise generators ("tinnitus instruments" or "combination instruments") may be more suitable than hearing aids alone. For these hearing losses the hearing aid may not be able to amplify soft sounds enough to interact with the tinnitus. In these cases masking noise from the built-in sound generator replaces ambient sound as the best means to reduce tinnitus audibility in quiet. Some clinicians recommend combination aids whenever tinnitus accompanies hearing loss. I prefer to try hearing aids first as there are a much greater range of devices and they feature the latest technology to improve hearing the most.

Sometimes tinnitus accompanies a total loss of hearing in just one ear, known as a "dead" ear. Using sound in a dead ear to mask tinnitus does not work; however, all is not lost! As mentioned earlier, tinnitus in one ear can sometimes be masked or reduced by sound in the opposite ear. So a masker can be fitted to the hearing ear and this sometimes helps the tinnitus.

For large hearing losses affecting both ears, sound therapy of any kind becomes difficult; even amplified sounds may not be loud enough to be heard. With such significant hearing losses, cochlear implants might assist hearing and result in some tinnitus relief by electrical stimulation of the hearing nerve. A cochlear implant ("bionic ear") consists of an array of small electrical stimulators arranged along a fine wire probe that is surgically implanted in the inner ear. Like a hearing aid, sound is picked up by a microphone and processed, but unlike a hearing aid which amplifies sound, the cochlear implant directly stimulates the auditory nerve. The implant transfers small electrical impulses which signal the frequency and timing of sound. The brain then needs to learn how these signals relate to speech and other important sounds. As a general rule cochlear implants are used when hearing aids offer limited benefit. Cochlear implants do reduce tinnitus in some cases. The electrical stimulation may directly interfere with the tinnitus generation or they may work the same way that hearing aids do—by keeping the auditory system busy with listening to sound other than the tinnitus. Your audiologist or physician should be able to advise you whether a cochlear implant is a viable option.

## Music as Therapy

"Music is the wine that fills the cup of silence."
R. Fripp

Music has been used as a therapeutic tool in the treatment of many clinical conditions by inducing a relaxation response or causing an attention shift away from problems. Music can result in muscle relaxation, slowing of heart rate and decrease in blood pressure leading to improved mood and reduction in effects of stress. It has also been successfully used to improve sleep and in hospitals to divert attention away from pain.

Listening to music is one of the most common and effective self-help tinnitus treatments. For the management of tinnitus music that induces positive feelings should be used. Music from a friend's funeral will not likely have the desired positive emotional affect! Typically, orchestral music is used for reducing tinnitus; however, any music can be tried, and for some people even hard rock might have a positive result. In a study conducted by Al-Jasim (1988), subjects chose their own masker from a selection of pure tones, narrow and wideband noises, relaxation tapes (soft music with speaker teaching the listener how to relax physically and mentally), or music. No mention was made of the levels used but preference was given to music (87.8%), followed by relaxation tapes (7.3%), no masker (4.9%) and pure tones (0%).

When tinnitus is severe, attention-capturing music can be beneficial. For long-term tinnitus habituation to tinnitus, music which induces relaxation while reducing tinnitus audibility should be considered. I think music should be played at a low level whereby the music begins to blend with the tinnitus. Low-level music played in the background during quiet situations can help to draw attention away from the tinnitus. In choosing music the following ideas may prove helpful (Hann et al., in press):

- only music evoking positive feelings should be used;
- use music without vocals;
- use music without a pronounced bass beat; choose music that is pleasant but not too interesting or compelling;
- for short-term relief when tinnitus is severe, attention-capturing music can be beneficial;
- for long-term tinnitus habituation, use music which in duces relaxation while reducing tinnitus audibility;
- music should be played at a low level (ideally, where the music begins to blend with the tinnitus).

Some "alternative" music-based sound therapies claim to provide benefit not only for tinnitus but for problems as diverse as, stress, low energy, learning difficulties, attention deficit disorder, speech problems, auditory processing, dyslexia, autism, Down's Syndrome, depression, headaches, poor memory and concentration. These methods use electronically filtered musical recordings and are listened to at home for short periods every day. The rationale and claims made

for these therapies have not been scientifically validated. Any benefit in treating tinnitus probably occurs in the same way as normal
music.

## Stimulation of Deprived Areas of the Brain

"The human brain is unique in that it is the only container
of which it can be said that the more you put into it, the more
it will hold."

G. Doman

The parts of the brain involved in analyzing sound are organized
in a pitch by pitch manner know as a *tonotopic map*. The tonotopic
map is one way the brain codes sound. Each pitch of sound "maps"
to a specific area of the brain. You can imagine this map as being
much like a piano keyboard, arranged from low to high notes in a se-
quential manner. When damage occurs to a specific region of the
inner ear there's changed neural input to the corresponding region
of the brain. One theory suggests that the brain "turns up" it's internal "volume control" in response to changes in the outflow of activity from the ear. This in turn results in a change in responsiveness
or excitability in the auditory regions of the brain - causing tinnitus.
It has also been suggested by a number of researchers that when a
specific frequency region of the inner ear is injured (for example, a
high frequency hearing loss), the regions of the brain representing
adjacent frequencies expand so that frequencies neighboring the
damage become over-represented. This is like some keys being removed from the piano and the neighboring keys being made wider to
fill the missing space. It's suggested that this leads to over-activity
in the expanded regions and tinnitus results as a consequence of this.

It's believed that the over-activity might be reversed by driving
the system with sound. Sound generators or hearing aids deliver a
low level of sound to the ear which causes the auditory nerve fibers
to fire at a faster rate than normal. This increase in activity reduces
the contrast between normal nerve activity and the tinnitus. With
prolonged persistent exposure to sound, the neural circuits may
change and reduce their response to tinnitus. Alternatively, researchers have been investigating the possibility that tinnitus may
be reduced by learning to discriminate between tinnitus and real
sounds. This exercise may raise activity in areas of the tonotopic map
neighboring tinnitus and in so doing reorganize the auditory cortex

so that the tinnitus activity is less prominent. This is in contrast to conventional use of broadband sound used in masking- or habituation-based therapies in which tinnitus sufferers are instructed not to attend to the tinnitus or the masking sound. New sound therapies may develop once this process is more fully understood.

## Devices

"Everybody has their taste in noises as well as in other matters."
J. Austen

There are a multitude of different devices available to provide sound therapy. Some of the more popular are outlined below.

### Hearing Aids

This was previously discussed. Hearing aids come in all shapes and sizes. They should be chosen on the basis of comfort and ability to partially mask tinnitus. Hearing aids are an excellent starting point to reduce tinnitus accompanying hearing loss. Seek out an audiologist who understands tinnitus.

### Tinnitus Masker

A *tinnitus masker* or sound generator is a small noise maker resembling a hearing aid, which can be worn on or in the ear and produces a sound of variable intensity and frequency.

### Combination Instrument

*Combination instruments* combine a hearing aid with a built-in tinnitus masker. They're available from a limited number of hearing aid manufacturers. Consult your hearing healthcare practitioner.

### Assistive Listening Devices

Assistive listening devices are used in conjunction with hearing aids. FM radio aids, infrared and loop systems can used to implement acoustic therapy. A FM or loop system connected to a radio or any sound-producing device can transmit sound to headphones or hearing aids.

## Desktop Devices

Desktop devices are designed to produce a limited, but variety of different sounds. Usually, there's a choice of a number of nature sounds (for example, surf, rain, waterfalls). They're used at home to enhance the sound environment and can be used in conjunction with hearing aids. Nighttime is often a time of the day that tinnitus sufferers dread because of the quietness of the bedroom and the loudness of the tinnitus. Desktop devices can be left on throughout the night to provide constant stimulation. Rather than tinnitus being the first thing heard on awakening you hear the sound from the bedside device, a much better way to start the day! Some of these devices are combined with alarm clocks; others work with headphones or "pillow speakers" to avoid disturbing anyone else in the room.

## Sounds Produced by Computer Programs

Masking and complex sound software is available to download from the Internet. This software uses the sound card on your computer to generate a variety of different sounds and enables you to choose the pitch and loudness of the masking sound. Various sounds selected from music, nature sounds, and broadband noise can be downloaded. It's an easy way to obtain masking sounds to listen to.

## Sound Recording and Playback Systems

A number of companies market prerecorded sounds. Compact discs (CDs) containing relaxing background music can be purchased and played on a portable or installed playback system. These can be a useful alternative to desktop devices. A good selection of music on CD can be very helpful to divert attention from tinnitus on quiet days around the house. MP3 players can be used much in the same way as sound generators or a CD player.

## Radio

"Talk Radio" is not usually recommended, as it's unlikely to reduce stress. A radio tuned between radio stations produces a fairly good masking sound. Listening to music is also a good masking option. However, in all of the choices you have limited control over what sound you will hear in the ensuing minutes.

## Cochlear Implants

As discussed earlier, cochlear implants are surgically implanted prosthetic devices which overcome hearing loss by directly stimulating the hearing nerve. These are usually an option for managing tinnitus when it's paired with a severe hearing loss.

## Special Modified Sound Approaches

> "When we talk about understanding, surely it takes place only when the mind listens completely - the mind being your heart, your nerves, your ears - when you give your whole attention to it."
>
> J. Krishnamutri

### Production of Residual Inhibition

Some clinicians believe that long-term residual inhibition can be accomplished by listening to sounds closely resembling tinnitus. The sounds are matched using computer software and then recorded to CD or onto an MP3 player. The length and extent of residual inhibition is difficult to predict for an individual and may last from seconds to hours and rarely days. There's considerable research interest in how this residual inhibition effect may be made to last longer.

### Using a Narrowband Centered on the Tinnitus

Masking with sound centered at tinnitus pitch has been suggested as an alternative to broadband sound. The idea is that a sound at tinnitus pitch can be effective at masking while interfering less with important sounds—such as speech. However, some people find narrowband sounds annoying and consequently most masking and habituation treatments use broadband sounds.

### High Frequency Stimulation

Other researchers believe that very high frequency (10-20 kHz) stimulation might benefit tinnitus. This could be accomplished by using "ultrasonic bone vibration" or by a high-fidelity miniature sound generator. There's limited evidence for its efficacy.

## Canceling Tinnitus with an Acoustic Signal

Several people have noted over the years that if tinnitus was a sine wave, it could be completely canceled (and eliminated from perception) if you could add in an acoustical signal of the exact same frequency and intensity, but opposite phase. *Noise* or *phase cancellation* headphones in industry and as used on aircraft can be successful in reducing the effects of background noise. However, tinnitus is not a sound. It's a signal within the neural pathways, and so does not have phase, so it cannot be canceled in this manner. In my opinion, this therapy probably achieves masking rather than cancellation.

## Combinations of Processed Sound

Of course there already are, and will continue to be new approaches that combine some of the above strategies. For example, one approach combines partial masking and processed music. The merits of the all sound therapies need to be fully explored in clinical trails. I suspect there will be some individual preferences; what works for one person will not suit another.

### Counseling to go with Sound Therapy

"The more alternatives, the more difficult the choice."
A' D'Allanival

Counseling should play an important role for almost every type of tinnitus treatment, particularly with use of sound therapy. Tinnitus counseling should be undertaken by an audiologist, physician or psychologist (see Chapter 1).

One very clear potential disadvantage of sound therapy devices is that they can be obtained from stores or over the Internet in the absence of appropriate medical, audiological or psychological evaluation. Remember that just putting on a sound therapy device is not going to cure your tinnitus. Sound therapy alone is not enough. If you're serious about reducing the effects of your tinnitus, the first step is seeing a clinician competent in tinnitus treatment. Self-help methods can follow once an understanding of the likely cause of tinnitus is achieved and any fears or worries have been dealt with.

# Summary

How does a person with tinnitus go about choosing which of the sound therapies mentioned is the right treatment option? It's unlikely that any single treatment is the best solution for everyone. It's important to consider whether the person with tinnitus has a hearing loss, their personality, lifestyle, treatment availability and cost. Choosing the best option is not straight forward, and is by no means a science. In my opinion, if there's a hearing loss, hearing aids should be the first option. If a hearing aid trial proves unsuccessful, sound therapy using music or noise should be tried. The potential effect of a noise generator can be estimated by listening to tinnitus with a shower running or water through a faucet. You can move closer or further away from the sound to change its level at your ear. If this "faucet test" makes the tinnitus less obvious, and the noise is not annoying, this may be an option. If the hissing sound is annoying or unhelpful, then relaxing music might be a better option. Some treatments require frequent visits to a clinic, so choosing a treatment offered in a nearby town is often desirable. Hearing aids, maskers and other devices can be expensive, but the benefits can far out weigh the costs. Finding a clinic and clinician that you can trust and feel understands tinnitus is critical.

Ultimately, success in defeating tinnitus rests with you. Tinnitus can and should be reduced by a combination of counseling and sound therapy, whichever option you choose you must give it your best shot for it to succeed.

# References

Tyler R. (2000) Psychoacoustical Measurement. In: Tyler RS (Ed.), <u>Tinnitus Handbook</u>. San Diego: Singular Publishing, pp. 181-203.

Henry JL, Wilson PH. (2002) <u>A Self-Management Guide for the Ringing in Your Ears</u>. Boston: Allyn and Bacon.

Saltzman M, Ersner M. (1947) A hearing aid for the relief of tinnitus aurium. *Laryngoscope* 57:358-366.

Feldmann H. (1971) Homolateral and contralateral masking of tinnitus by noise-bands and by pures tones. *Audiology*, 10(3), 138-144.

Schleuning AJ, Johnson RM, Vernon JA. (1980) Evaluation of a tinnitus masking program: a follow-up study of 598 patients. *Ear & Hearing* 1(2):71-74.

Worden FG. (1976) Auditory Habituation. In: Tighe TJ, Leaton RN, (Eds.) Habituation. New York: Erlbaum Associates, pp. 109-137.

Hallam RS, Rachman S, Hinchcliffe R. (1984) Psychological aspects of tinnitus. In: Rachman S, ed. Contributions to Medical Psychology. Oxford: Pergamon, 31-53.

Searchfield GD. (2006) Hearing aids and tinnitus In: Tyler RS (Ed.) Tinnitus Treatments. New York: Thieme.

Surr RK, Montgomery AA, Mueller HG. (1985) Effect of amplification on tinnitus among new hearing aid users. *Ear and Hearing* 6(2):71-75.

Al-Jassim AH. (1988) The use of Walkman Mini-stereo system as a tinnitus masker. *Journal of Laryngology and Otology* 102(1):27-8.

Hann D, Searchfield GD, Sanders M, Wise K. (In Press) Strategies for the selection of music in the short-term management of mild tinnitus.

CHAPTER ELEVEN

# What to Expect from Your Physician and Healthcare Professionals

## Tanit Ganz Sanchez, MD, PhD

*Tinnitus Research Group, University of São Paulo Medical School, Brazil*

**Dr. Sanchez** received her Medical Degree from the University of São Paulo in 1990. She is an otolaryngologist considered to be a "different doctor" because one-hundred percent of her professional life is now dedicated to tinnitus. She works motivating professionals and the public to be more involved in solutions to tinnitus. In 1994, she created the Tinnitus Research Group in the University of São Paulo. In 1999, she created the Brazilian Tinnitus Educational and Support Group, a network of philanthropy that will be operating in eight cities starting in 2008. In 2006, she published her first book for tinnitus patients and created the national Day of Tinnitus Consciousness - established as November 11th - in order to reach the public with updated information.

## Introduction

Tinnitus is a symptom and not a single disease! It might have one of many contributing causes. Additionally, people react quite differently to their tinnitus, and you probably have already noticed it. Two individuals with the same age and gender, the same degree of hearing loss, and even the same loudness of tinnitus, might have different causes. The identification of these different factors related to tinnitus is important in order to choose the adequate treatment. The complexity of tinnitus, as well as the complexity of our human nature, means that a wide range of healthcare professionals might be able to help. The management of tinnitus patients often demands a deep evaluation and treatment by a team of professionals. The otolaryngologist is the core physician of this team, and should act in accordance with the other professionals. This chapter reviews the roles of such professionals and what you should expect from each of them. I will suggest some information that would be helpful to prepare you before visiting them.

## Documenting your History in Preparation for your Appointment

Your healthcare professional who you decide to ask for help will need as many clues as possible. All information about your tinnitus is important, even the details. This includes:

- when your tinnitus first began;
- what your tinnitus sounds like (for example, buzzing, humming, a waterfall, heartbeat);
- what you think caused your tinnitus;
- what makes your tinnitus better or worse;
- whether your tinnitus affects your emotional well-being, hearing, sleep or concentration;
- whether your tinnitus affects your work or social interations;
- what treatments you have tried for tinnitus;
- if you have a hearing loss, when it first began;
- whether your hearing loss fluctuates;
- whether you are bothered by loud sounds;
- whether you have ever been exposed to loud noise;
- whether you have balance problems;
- what medications and/or supplements you are taking for tinnitus (make a list);
- what medications and/or supplements you are taking for other ailments (make a list).

In addition to these items, information about your general health history is also important to understand your tinnitus in the wider context of your overall health. The information that will be helpful will include:

- your occupation;
- other diseases or general health problems that you have (for example, diabetes, hyper- or hypothyroidism, lipid disorders, hearing loss, migraines);
- whether you have jaw or neck discomfort or pain;
- your present and past smoking and alcohol use;
- unusual eating/drinking habits, such as overuse of caffeine, fats and sweets/candies or prolonged fasting periods;
- family history of diseases (for example, diabetes mellitus, hearing loss, autoimmune diseases—when the immune system attacks itself).

## Questions You Should Ask

Before you go to your appointment, you also might want to prepare a list of things you would like to ask. There might be some personal circumstances about your life that are important to share, or you might have some concerns that are important for you. Don't lose the opportunity to ask questions, but please be as concise as you can to make the interview as efficient as possible.

## Your Physician

Physicians are trained in medicine to diagnose and treat health conditions throughout your body. They provide prescription of medications and can perform surgery that should be needed. A general practitioner focuses on general healthcare. The physician who concentrates on your ears, nose and throat is called an *otolaryngologist*. Those that specialize in the ear are referred to as an *otologist*. The otolaryngologist must identify all the different factors that might be related to your tinnitus and provide a diagnosis. The identification of each of these factors related to your tinnitus could be a key point for the success of the treatment.

Although usually not the case, your tinnitus might be related to some other illness. If the other illness is treated, your tinnitus might improve. The factors that might indirectly affect the ear or the brain include *metabolic* (disturbances in processes involved in providing energy and maintaining the functions of cells and systems throughout the body), *pharmacological* (when some medicines and drugs influence your tinnitus), *cardiovascular* (when heart and blood vessels are involved), *neurological*, dental and psychological diseases. In some special cases, vascular and muscular structures related to the head and neck region might be involved. There might even be more than one possible cause or factor related to the tinnitus. Keep in mind that the identification of such factors or combination of factors in your case is fundamental for choosing the best treatment and for the success of therapy. So, the physician is a detective, trying to gather enough clues to find "which factors might be guilty."

## The Interview and Clinical History

Although the evidence is sometimes weak linking these factors cited in the previous section to tinnitus in large and controlled surveys, they might be very important when you see the issue from an individual point of view. Thus, we usually ask patients whether they overuse caffeine or sweets/candies or fats in daily meals, whether they often undergo prolonged fasting periods, and whether they have family history of diabetes and high levels of fat in the blood. The fats are carried out in the blood in particles called *lipoproteins*, which are classified according to their density into very low-density lipoprotein; low-density lipoprotein and high-density lipoprotein. Studies have demonstrated that the higher the level of low-density lipoprotein cholesterol, the greater the risk of some heart and brain diseases, which may have implications for tinnitus.

During this detailed interview, your physician is performing a differential diagnosis to check some possibilities and to discard others (see Chapters 2, 3, and 7).

## Potential Causes of Tinnitus

### Auditory System Causes

First of all, the physician will likely look for wax or any disease in the external ear canal and the condition of the eardrum. The doctor will then examine your middle ear by looking for acute or chronic *otitis media* (when infection of the middle ear persists with pus discharge, potentially leading to middle ear damage and eardrum perforation), *tympanosclerosis* (a scarring of the eardrum caused by previous inflammation or infection, leading to hearing loss) or any sign of *otosclerosis* (condition in which abnormal bone grows keeping the *stapes* from moving, causing hearing loss). The audiological examination and *audiogram* (see below) will help to confirm if there's a middle or inner ear hearing loss. There can be fluid behind the eardrum, or fixation of the small bones (*ossicles*) of middle ear.

Inner ear causes are also to be considered. In patients over 60 years with a gradual high frequency hearing loss and without other likely causes present, the diagnosis is usually *presbycusis* (the natural aging of the ear), although other problems might be involved. With a history of noise exposure and a *notched audiogram* around

4000 Hz, the likely diagnosis is noise-induced tinnitus. Other causes can be: *Ménière's disease* (combines sporadic attacks of tinnitus, hearing loss, sensation of ear fullness and dizziness), *acoustic schwannoma* (benign tumor of the vestibular nerve), severe head or neck injury or post infection (for example, *meningitis*).

## Metabolic Causes

Metabolic causes (defined above) are involved in some patients with overuse of caffeine (coffee, black tea or malt, chocolate, and most cola drinks), disturbance of carbohydrate or lipids metabolism, or deficiency of zinc. It is important to consider these factors because they represent tinnitus that can be treated in some patients. The inner ear has a dense group of blood vessels. The better your blood vessels are working, the better your chance to have healthy hearing and balance.

## Pharmacological Causes

Many drugs can worsen or produce tinnitus as a side effect in some patients, including *salicylates, aminoglycoside antibiotics, diuretics* and *chemotherapy agents.* In such cases, tinnitus might be relieved if the drug can be discontinued early; however, you need to ask your physician first! Usually, it's important to make these decisions as soon as possible.

## Cardiovascular Causes

The inner ear is irrigated by one single and small artery, and there are no additional sources of blood circulation (as there is in the heart or brain after obstruction of the *artery lumen*). Thus, it's easy to understand why cardiovascular diseases can affect this artery and cause ear problems, including tinnitus. Some examples are blood *hypertension,* heart failure, *anemia, peripheral vascular failure,* and so forth. In such cases, we should always control the underlying disease.

## Neurological Causes

Diseases that affect the central and/or peripheral nervous system can also cause tinnitus. This could be a result of severe head injury, cerebral vascular accident, infectious central nervous system diseases such as *meningitis, multiple sclerosis* (a neurologic disorder of unknown cause; widespread disease may affect auditory pathway), and *whiplash* (sudden flexion and extension movement of the cervical spine caused by car accidents).

## Dental Causes

The association between tinnitus and dental/jaw muscle function is controversial. The *temporomandibular joint* connects the jaw to the skull. Its dysfunction may have local causes (dental loss, strong biting, asymmetric growth, and trauma). If there's no other obvious cause of the tinnitus, and if there's dental or jaw pain, you might be referred for a dental assessment.

## Psychological Causes

You might also be asked if you experience anxiety, depression or panic attacks. Even if these problems are not the origin of tinnitus, they might contribute to your reaction to the tinnitus (see Chapters 4 and 5). In troublesome cases, you might be referred to a psychiatrist or psychologist. Your personality skills, previous experiences and personal beliefs about tinnitus have much to do with the way you experience and react to your tinnitus.

## Physical Examination

A complete physical examination is recommended, checking up your general health, blood circulation, the respiratory tract (nose, throat, larynx, trachea, bronchi, and lungs) and the nervous system. The otolaryngology physical examination comprises the ear, nose, throat and neck parts. However, when tinnitus is the main complaint, the physical examination is often normal.

## Laboratory Tests

Laboratory tests are performed by analysis of the blood. They're helpful for screening some underlying health conditions that might influence your tinnitus pattern. The laboratory tests that might be ordered for all tinnitus patients might include the following:

**A blood cell count** to check for *anemia* or an excess of red blood cells (maybe a sign of poor blood circulation and oxygenation of inner ear cells).

**A fasting glucose test** is important to rule out *diabetes mellitus* (high blood glucose levels due to inability to metabolize carbohydrates) or pre-diabetes (a great tendency to develop diabetes because the blood glucose levels are higher than normal but not high enough to be identified as diabetes). In patients who report eagerness to eat sweets and prolonged fast periods, it's important to order a test to check for glucose and insulin levels before and after a meal. A high concentration of insulin or low concentration of glucose might compromise the active transportation of sodium and potassium in the inner ear.

**Lipid levels** (levels of fats in the blood) should be checked since some kind of *lipids* can worsen blood circulation.

**Thyroid hormone levels** evaluating for hyper- and hypothyroidism should be considered. The thyroid gland is located in the neck, and responsible for secretion of hormones for growth and metabolism. In hyperthyroidism there's overproduction of such hormones and their levels in the blood are high. In hypothyroidism, insufficient hormone is produced which is also a risk factor for high cholesterol levels.

**Serum zinc** is ordered mainly for the elderly, vegetarians, and individuals with nutritional deficiency (for example, after surgery to reduce the stomach). Zinc is present within the cells that play an important role in the body functioning and in the immune system. Zinc is also important in the central nervous system and in the auditory system.

**Serum reactions to syphilis** - *syphilis* is usually sexually transmitted and caused by a bacteria. It can cause serious injury not only to the unborn baby (congenital syphilis) but also to the adults (acquired syphilis). Both types can damage the inner ear, causing tinnitus.


### Imaging Studies

Imaging studies are an attempt to take a picture somewhere inside your body. Your medical assessment for tinnitus might include one or more of the following:

**Computed Tomography (CT scan)** is basically ordered to evaluate the bony structures in the ear. It's also useful to study the vessel alterations in pulsatile tinnitus.
**Magnetic Resonance Imaging (MRI)** provides highly detailed images of soft tissue structures in the ear and presence of tumors.

Some more recent imaging exams are referred to as *functional imaging*. These show, in a dynamic way, the more activate areas in the brain. Functional exams include the following:

**SPECT** (single photon emission computed tomography) is a special type of CT scan that can give information about blood flow and metabolism of tissues. A small amount of a radioactive material is injected into a vein and a scanner is used to make detailed images of areas inside the body where that radioactive substance is taken up by the cells.
**PET** (positron emission tomography) is based on the acquirement of body images by detection of the radiation from emission of positrons (tiny particles emitted from a radioactive material). It's also called PET scan.
**fMRI** (functional magnetic resonance imaging) is a noninvasive imaging test that uses magnetic resonance imaging to measure metabolic changes that take place in the part of the brain that is being used during particular cerebral tasks.

These imaging exams are used to view the structure and function of different areas of the brain, usually to search for abnormal blood flow or tumors. In the future, they might be used to evaluate or help determine different tinnitus subgroups, and to help direct treatment.

## Referrals to Other Physicians

There is a variety of medical specialties and the role they might play in helping the tinnitus patient. In some cases, psychiatrists are also indicated for controlling some disorders that are commonly present in tinnitus patients, such as anxiety and depression.

*Otolaryngologist* - makes a detailed medical evaluation, prescribes medications and performs ear, nose, throat and head and neck surgery. He or she also directs the involved medical team, checking which of the illnesses detected might be involved with your tinnitus.

*Neurologist* - makes the identification and control of associated neurological disorders. The neurologist chooses the best drug for these diseases avoiding those that can cause or worsen tinnitus complaint is fundamental.

*Endocrinologist* - controls associated endocrine diseases (endocrine glands and their hormone release) such as diabetes mellitus, pre-diabetes, increase in blood lipids and hyper- or hypothyroidism.

*Rheumatologist* - assesses and treats musculoskeletal disorders including chronic arthritis, degenerative and autoimmune diseases, inflammations of blood vessels in the body. This professional evaluation is useful in cases of rapidly progressive hearing loss and Ménière's disease.

*Neurosurgeon* - is always indicated when surgery on the brain, spine, and other parts of the nervous system is mandatory.

*Psychiatrist* - identifies associated psychiatric disorders and controls some disorders that are commonly present in tinnitus patients, such as anxiety, stress, and mood disorders (depression and mania).

## Your Audiologist

Audiologists are trained in hearing disorders, including hearing loss, balance problems and tinnitus. They also often play a key role in diagnosis and treatment since they measure hearing loss and tinnitus, and provide hearing and tinnitus counseling and devices.

### Measuring your Hearing

Some of the tests done by an audiologist include the following:

**Pure-tone audiometry** which measures your ability to hear the lowest intensity tone for different tone frequencies.

**Loudness Discomfort Level** measures the levels at which sounds become uncomfortable. This is the test used to evaluate individuals with *hyperacusis* (see Chapter 13).

**Otoacoustic Emissions** is an exam that measures sounds produced in the cochlea and presumably relates to the functioning of the outer hair cells (see Chapter 7). It is widely used as a screening tool for hearing loss in newborns, but can be helpful in some cases with normal hearing thresholds, central deafness or inconsistent responses to audiometry.

**Auditory Brainstem Response (ABR)** is a technique that measures electrical activity produced by the hearing system nerves within the brainstem in response to a brief sound. It provides a way of evaluating the presence of lesions in the auditory nerve or brainstem. It's often used in patients with asymmetric hearing loss or with unilateral or asymmetric tinnitus to search for the presence of tumors.

## Measuring your Tinnitus

Measuring tinnitus is one of the most difficult challenges an audiologist undertakes. This is because typically in the most common type of tinnitus (subjective) the internal sound is being measured against an external sound (from the audiometer). It often involves a certain amount of guesswork on the patient's part. Here are the two most important parameters audiologists consider during their assessment.

Tinnitus loudness is the level of a tone (from an audiometer) that can be adjusted so that it has the same loudness as your tinnitus. The resultant loudness match is often about 5-10 dB SL (decibels sensation level, that is, decibels higher than the minimum needed to hear the softest sounds). It is important to realize that sensation level is not a direct measure of loudness; it's a measure of the level of a sound above the threshold of hearing. Therefore, some patients who describe their tinnitus as very loud can have a low sensation level loudness match. However, if they have a hearing loss at the matched frequency, may report their tinnitus as being very soft. If they have a significant hearing loss at the frequency of the test signal, even a low sensation level tinnitus can appear quite loud.

Pitch matching is attained when the frequency of a tone can be adjusted (such as on an audiometer) so that it has the same pitch as the most prominent pitch of your tinnitus. Even though tinnitus quality might include several sounds (for example, a buzz and a tone), most patients can choose a most prominent pitch.

## Your Psychologist

Psychologists are trained in understanding and treating human behavior. Psychological therapies are often helpful in more troublesome cases of tinnitus.

Standardized psychological tests are usually used in tinnitus patients with some degree of anxiety, depression and sleep disorders. Clinical interview might be interesting in these cases. The treatment is chosen according to different lines of thoughts (see Chapters 4-6).

## Other Healthcare Professionals

There are other healthcare professionals that can be helpful for the evaluation and treatment of tinnitus.

A *physiotherapist* can be helpful in some special cases with associated head and neck pain and modulation of tinnitus patterns by movements of the head and neck. This practitioner heals the body through physical methods such as massages and exercises.

The *dentist* specializes in the treatment of teeth and temporomandibular joint diseases.

The *nutritionist* can be consulted for patients with hypertension, high levels of cholesterol and triglyceride, and glucose disorders. This practitioner is an expert on foods, vitamins and nutrients.

## Medications for Tinnitus

There are a variety of treatments available for tinnitus patients when a specific cause is recognized. You may have already tried some of the following in an effort to resolve the problem. I'll close this chapter with a brief discussion of the more commonly applied treatments.

### Outer Ear Medications

Excessive amount of wax blocking the ear canal or loose hairs (or fragments of skin peeled off from the ear canal) touching the *tympanic membrane* may cause tinnitus. In such cases, clearing the external ear canal with water irrigation or with small instruments may provide immediate relief. Your otolaryngologist will choose the best way to do it. <u>Never</u> try to do it by yourself, for example, by going to the drugstore or even by *ear coning* (also called ear candling) which can permanently destroy or damage parts of the ear!

## Middle Ear Medications

Some middle ear problems such as infections (*otitis*) and muscle contractions (either of *tensor tympani* or *stapedius,* the two tiny muscles of the middle ear) can be associated with your tinnitus and may be transient. If controlled, tinnitus can resolve adequately.

When middle ear muscle contractions are involved, muscle relaxant drugs, *benzodiazepines* (minor tranquilizers that act primarily upon the central nervous system) and anticonvulsant drugs (or "antiepileptic" drugs, used to suppress the excessive function of central nervous system cells) can be prescribed.

Middle ear infections can be treated mostly by antibiotic and anti-inflammatory drugs. In some cases, eardrops may be necessary.

## Medications Affecting Blood Flow

The special anatomy and physiology of the inner ear and the central auditory system (see Chapter 7) can explain why some medications acting in the blood flow are useful for improving your tinnitus (see also Chapter 12). They're usually called *vasodilators* drugs (betahistine, cinnarizine, flunarizin, piracetam, papaverine, nimodipine, Ginkgo biloba among others) or *hemorrheologic agents* (drugs that improve blood flow changing the red blood cell properties, such as pentoxifilin). They're used in order to ameliorate the cochlear and brain functions by increasing tissue oxygenation and nutrition.

Other types of drugs *(corticosteroids, diuretics)* can be used alone or in association to medications affecting the blood flow to treat some special entities such as sudden deafness, noise trauma and Ménière's disease.

## Medications for Sleep, Anxiety and Depression

Anxiety, depression or panic attacks might contribute to a strong and negative reaction to tinnitus (see above and Chapters 4 and 5). The benzodiazepines (see also Chapter 12) are useful in treating associated anxiety, insomnia, agitation, seizures and muscle spasms (such as *myoclonus,* see chapter 2). The use of benzodiazepine should only commence after medical consultation, and in the smallest dosage possible to provide an acceptable level of symptom relief. Unfortunately, dependence is an undesirable sideeffect.

Antidepressant agents are indicated for associated depression and hyperacusis (see Chapter 12). There are many types of antidepressants.

## Surgical Considerations

### Middle Ear Surgery

As a general rule, surgical treatments are indicated when clinical management fails. However, just a few causes of tinnitus are suitable for surgery, and they're usually linked to middle ear problems. Some examples where surgery might be used to treat tinnitus include: chronic infections, eardrum perforation, disruption of the three tiny bones of the middle ear, middle ear muscle contractions and otosclerosis (see Chapter 2). In all these cases, tinnitus relief might be provided.

### Surgery of the Acoustic Nerve, Brainstem, and Brain

The presence of auditory or brain tumors (even when benign) or vascular loops (when a blood vessel touches and compresses the auditory nerve) usually requires surgical treatment. The surgery in these cases is more complex, and of course there are associated risks, most commonly, sacrificing hearing in the operated ear. Your physician will advise you on the best treatment options.

## Changing your Diet

Feeling well is strongly related to the treatment and prevention of many health disorders. Eating healthy foods and regular exercise is good for all of us. For tinnitus, it might be interesting to try some "therapeutic tests" to check whether changing your diet reduces the loudness or discomfort of your tinnitus.

Some patients do especially well when they reduce the levels of caffeine intake (coffee, black tea, chocolate and drinks) for one week as a therapeutic test. However, coffee might have different concentration of caffeine in different countries and this should be taken into consideration. Others have reported that their tinnitus is minimized with a 30-day diet reducing sugar. Lastly, reversing the high levels of blood lipids may be interesting for tinnitus improvement, especially in cases in which such alterations are recent. This can be done by reducing oil, butter, fatty meals (including full cream or whole milk and fatty meats), fried and fast foods. It's also important to eat at least 5 or 6 times a day (period of 3 or 4 hours) and keeping away from sugar, sweets and candies.

### Transcranial Magnetic Stimulation

There have been some recent reports of short-term reduction of tinnitus with repetitive *Transcranial Magnetic Stimulation*. A non-published study has just suggested that the reduction of tinnitus obtained by this method in normal hearing patients - a rare subgroup of tinnitus patients - may be stable up to 6 months after treatment. However, this approach is still considered experimental at this time.

### Hearing Aids

Most tinnitus patients have a hearing loss, and will benefit from a hearing aid. Hearing aids often help tinnitus by means of total or partial *masking* (see Chapter 10).

### Counseling

There are a variety of counseling procedures available to help tinnitus patients. Different specialists may provide tinnitus counseling, including audiologists, psychologists and physicians. But they need to be knowledgeable about tinnitus and counseling to achieve such a task. It's a really important step for you to understand your problem and be motivated to participate in achieving the best results.

### Sound Therapy

Many tinnitus patients report their tinnitus is less prominent in the presence of background sound, such as broadband noise or music.

Wearable devices to mask or *habituate* tinnitus are also available (see Chapter 10).

## Conclusions

Tinnitus is a multifaceted symptom, and there are many healthcare professionals who can play an important role in helping you with your tinnitus.

Your physician will perform a medical examination. You will most likely see an otolaryngologist or otologist. You should expect a thorough clinical history, and possibly laboratory tests or imaging studies. An audiologist will measure your hearing and tinnitus. If appropriate, they might also provide counseling, and fit hearing aids or tinnitus devices. A psychologist can provide counseling, particularly in more severe cases.

Unfortunately, in most situations, there's no cure for tinnitus. However, many patients do improve with adequate treatment adapted for each particular case. There may be some diseases that can be treated by a physician. If you have a hearing loss, an audiologist can provide you with hearing aids to help you to hear better and also improve your tinnitus (by means of environmental sounds covering it up—masking it). A psychologist can help provide counseling in more severe cases.

Remember that patients and professionals need to be a team. So, you're also a critical part of this team. You have to do your part in this job, too. It's important that you play an active role in providing important information about your health history, and also that you keep positive and hopeful that you'll improve. You also are a key participant in most treatments, particularly those that involve counseling and sound therapy.

# CHAPTER TWELVE

# Medications, Supplements and Alternative Medicines

## Claudia Barros Coelho, MD, PhD
*The University of Iowa, Iowa City*

---

**Dr. Coelho** pursued her medical degree from Fundação Faculdade Federal de Medicina de Porto Alegre and did her residency training in otolaryngology at Clinicas Hospital of Porto Alegre, both in Porto Alegre, Brazil. She completed her PhD at the Department of Otolaryngology from the University of São Paulo, Brazil. She divides her professional practice as an otolaryngologist in Brazil and as a research scientist at The Department of Otolaryngology and Head and Neck Surgery of The University of Iowa, Iowa City, Iowa. Her field of research is the study of tinnitus and hyperacusis in children and adults.

---

## Introduction

There is no medication or supplement that has been widely accepted (replicated in well-controlled studies) as a cure for tinnitus. There are many medications and supplements that can help with your reaction to tinnitus (for example, antidepressants and sleep medications). A few scientific studies on tinnitus treatments have reported that some tinnitus sufferers benefitted from medications and supplements. However, the appropriate studies have not been done to show which subgroups of tinnitus patients will benefit from which substances.

This scenario presents an unsatisfactory and perhaps confusing situation. It might be that there's a substance that will help you with your tinnitus. No one knows what medication or supplement might work for you, however. Therefore, some clinicians might suggest a substance, and many tinnitus sufferers try them. Some tinnitus sufferers might indeed be helped. However, the chance of being helped is quite low, and there are some risks. Some substances, even those not monitored by the *Food and Drug Administration* (FDA) can have serious negative side effects. Additionally, trying several substances that fail to show improvement can have a seriously negative outcome on one's emotional well-being. Additionally, the attention focused on finding the cure can be counterproductive to accepting and accommodating the tinnitus.

Having said this, it might be helpful for you to understand medications, supplements and alternative treatments, and how they relate, or might relate, to treatments. This chapter is organized in the following manner. First, I'll review classes of medications and describe a few specific medications that have been tried for tinnitus. Next, I'll review some "alternative treatments" that have been considered for treatments. Then I'll review some classes of medications that have been used to treat tinnitus reactions. I'll also mention drugs that might cause tinnitus. In rare cases, stopping the intake of these might eliminate your tinnitus. You'll not find me recommending a treatment to cure your tinnitus.

## Classes of Prescription Medications to Treat Tinnitus

Many medications have been studied to treat tinnitus. I'm going to describe them according to their probable mechanism of action. Some of them require special care and clinical follow up. For example, anticonvulsants and antidepressants require gradual increase in the dosage to reach adequate concentration. They also require a gradual decrease in the dosage at the end of treatment. This is because there are possible withdrawal symptoms which might occur, such as sleep loss, nausea, dizziness and headaches. This is why it's important to carefully titrate down your meds under medical supervision. Some general principles on drug therapy are described in Table 12-I.

## Oral Medications

### Drugs that Act on Blood Viscosity, Vasodilatation and Circulation

These drugs have an action of increasing blood circulation. This can be achieved by thinning the blood or dilating the blood vessels, thereby increasing their permeability (and thereby allowing blood nutrients to pass into nearby tissue). The rationale behind this application is to increase blood oxygen transport function in the auditory pathway. This might help if tinnitus is related to some areas of the cochlea and auditory nerve that might not be receiving enough oxygen. Some examples of this group of drugs includes pentoxifylline, trimetazidine, cyclandelate, nimodipine, flunarizine, betahistine, cinnarizine and eperisone.

Table 12-I : Some important concerns about medications

> • **Do not take any medication for your tinnitus before having an examination by a physician.**
>
> • **Do not change how you are supposed to take your prescription (increasing or decreasing the dosage or the frequency you are supposed to take it).**
>
> • **If you have adverse effects from your medication, talk to your physician before making any change.**
>
> • **Some people expect to have an immediate result from tinnitus treatments. Usually, a minimal period of time is expected until a medication might have an action your tinnitus.**
>
> • **Do not take any medication or supplement if you are pregnant or breastfeeding without your physician's approval.**
>
> • **Make sure your physician is aware of all the medications and supplements you are taking, both over-the-counter and prescription, herbal products and nutritional supplements.**

## Acamprosate

Acamprosate is a drug used for the treatment of alcohol dependence. A recent clinical trial has suggested efficacy to treat tinnitus in some patients. At the time of this writing, further studies are necessary to confirm this result.

## Drugs that Act on Neural Response

The targets of these drugs are neurotransmitters which are chemicals involved in the transmission of activity across nerve junctions (see Chapter 3). They act by modulating the activity and the efficiency of information on transmission across these junctions. Table 12-II represents a detailed explanation of how theses chemicals act.

Table 12 -II: Neurotransmitters—'what they are and how they act (also see Chapter 2)

---

• **Communication of information between neurons is done by the movement of chemicals across a small gap called synapse.**

• **These chemicals are called *neurotransmitters*. They are released from one neuron at the presynaptic nerve terminal.**

• **When these chemicals cross the synapse, they may be accepted by the next neuron in a special place called receptor.**

• **The activity on the receptor site may lead to an action on this neuron that can be either excitatory or inhibitory.**

---

### *Anticonvulsants*

These drugs are primarily used to prevent seizures or control their incidence or severity. Some are considered "versatile" and are used for a variety of other disorders, including tinnitus. Carbamazepine, lamotrigine and gabapentine are examples of these drugs that have been used to treat tinnitus. They're usually prescribed when other types of medications fail. The side effects of anticonvulsant medications are generally mild (drowsiness, hair loss, nausea, tremor, and weight gain). Occasionally, more serious side effects occur, such as liver problems and ovarian cysts.

### *Benzodiazepines*

Benzodiazepines are a class of drugs that have a tranquillizer effect, promote sleep, muscle relaxation and also have anticonvulsant properties. Their varieties of effects are promoted by modulating the activity of GABA (gamma-aminobutyric acid) receptor. GABA is a chemical in the brain that is found at many levels of the central auditory pathway. Changes on its action might be related to tinnitus (see Chapter 3). Medications such as alprazolam clonazepam, diazepam, flurazepam and oxazepam are included in this family of drugs. Some long-term effects deserve special attention, especially the risk of dependency and withdrawal symptoms upon discontinuation or dosage reduction.

### Selective Serotonin Reuptake Inhibitors

These drugs work by preventing the reuptake (reabsorption) of serotonin, one of the brain chemicals thought to cause depression. This action increases the level of serotonin in the brain. This family of drugs includes citalopram, escitalopram, fluoxetine, paroxetine and sertraline. They have been successfully used to treat tinnitus in some patients with and without depressive symptoms. The basis for this therapy is thought to rely on the interplay between non-auditory brainstem structures and the central auditory pathways.

### Tricyclic Antidepressants

This class of drugs blocks the reuptake (reabsorption) of certain chemicals in the brain such as norepinephrine (noradrenaline) and serotonin. They present antidepressant and analgesic effects. Trimipramine, nortriptyline and amitriptyline have been used to treat tinnitus. Amitriptyline has demonstrated to be more effective especially for patients with severe tinnitus accompanied by sleep disturbance.

### Blood Vessel Injection Medication

#### Anesthetics

Lidocaine is a local anesthetic (similar to those used in dental treatments) and several studies have suggested that tinnitus might be relieved in some patients. It acts on neuronal pathways responsible for the generation of tinnitus, similar to its action on pain pathways. Because of its short-term effect on tinnitus and possible serious adverse effects, it has been abandoned in clinical practice.

## *Medications Injected through the Eardrum*

It's also possible to deliver medication directly into the middle ear. It's done through a minimal surgical procedure. Some medications, such as *lidocaine, caroverine, steroids* and *gentamicin* have been studied to treat tinnitus using injections through the eardrum.

Lidocaine was shown to be effective in decreasing tinnitus in some, but most otologists have abandoned it. Relief was only temporary and the presence of side effects was severe (vertigo, nausea, vomiting).

Caroverine is a glutamate antagonist (acts by inhibiting glutamate activity). Glutamate is the major excitatory neurotransmitter in the brain. Excess of this chemical in the cochlea can be toxic to the inner hair cells. With its use, some researchers have observed reduction on some types of tinnitus associated with noise exposure, ototoxic drugs and Ménière's disease.

Gentamicin (an antibiotic) has been shown to eliminate or reduce tinnitus in some patients with Ménière's disease. It can only be used in patients with no serviceable hearing because it is toxic to the cochlea, causing hearing loss.

*Corticosteroid* application has helped some tinnitus patients and has few side effects.

## Alternative Treatments

Alternative treatments are a group of healthcare practices and products that are not presently considered to be part of conventional medicine. Although some of theses therapies have shown some scientific evidence of benefit, most of them still require well-designed scientific studies to determine their effectiveness, evaluate their safety and discover their action on diseases for which they're used. Some of the more frequently used alternative treatments for tinnitus are described next. (For more information on alternative treatments, go to http://nccam.nih.gov/health/whatiscam/.)

### Acupuncture

*Acupuncture* has been used in China for more than 2,000 years, being one of the oldest and most commonly used medical procedures in the world. According to traditional Chinese medicine, health is achieved by maintaining the body in a "balanced state." Diseases are thought to be due to an internal imbalance. In order to maintain the body in balance, a procedure involving stimulation of anatomical points called acupuncture points (there are more than 2,000 points on the body) are used. The point is penetrated into the skin with a thin, solid, metallic needle that's manipulated by the hands or by electrical stimulation.

It's proposed that acupuncture produces its effects regulating the central nervous system through changes in brain chemicals. (To find more detailed information you might consider the following website: http://nccam.nih.gov/health/acupuncture/)

Clinical trials have failed to demonstrate that acupuncture is effective to treat tinnitus. Nevertheless, some patients have mentioned a decrease in tension and improved sleep. You might experience minimal pain as the acupuncture needles are inserted. If they're inserted improperly or if you make movements, you can feel soreness and pain during the treatment. People who take this kind of alternative treatment should take some safety precautions to avoid contamination and infections. I recommend the use of disposable needles taken from a sealed package as well as disinfection of treatments sites with alcohol or another disinfectant before inserting the needles.

## Hyperbaric Oxygen Therapy

*Hyperbaric oxygen therapy* consists of breathing pure oxygen in a special chamber. It has been used in patients who develop hearing loss and tinnitus after a sudden hearing loss. The rationale is to increase the supply of oxygen to the ear and brain to reduce the severity of hearing loss and tinnitus. A recent review has suggested that there's insufficient evidence to determine if it's helpful for tinnitus or not.

## Dietary Supplements

A *dietary supplement* is a product taken by mouth that contains an ingredient intended to supplement the diet. Dietary ingredients might include vitamins, minerals, herbs or other botanicals, amino acids, and substances such as enzymes. Their use has become very popular. Estimates are that approximately 40% of all Americans take some form of a dietary supplement. Many tinnitus patients are among them. Although they're often identified as "natural," they can cause terrible side effects and most are not regulated. Before consuming these substances you should be aware of some concerns described in Table 12-III. Natural remedies are not always safe.

Some of the more common supplements that have been tried for tinnitus will be discussed next.

Table 12-III: Concerns about natural remedies

> • Herbs and nutritional supplements are not always safe, even when they are labeled "natural."
> • Their contents are standardized and might have different degrees of purity, strength, effect and could be contaminated.
> • The FDA does not inspect or regulate natural remedies the way they do for prescription drugs.
> • They affect your body and could interact with prescription medicines that you take.

### Ginkgo biloba

*Ginkgo biloba* is the world's oldest living tree species. Extracts of ginkgo leaves have been used for medicinal purposes for at least 5000 years in China. Ginkgo has been most widely prescribed as a treatment for *peripheral vascular disease* (insufficient blood flow to the limbs because of damage to blood vessels) and *cerebral insufficiency* (not enough blood reaching the brain) causing concentration difficulties, loss of memory, dizziness and tinnitus.

Ginkgo might influence tinnitus by increasing inner ear and cerebral blood circulation and protection against free radicals. Several investigators have studied its use on tinnitus, but the results are conflicting; positive on some, but no effect on others.

Some authorities recommended that you should not take ginkgo if you have seizures (as in epilepsy) or a bleeding disorder. They also recommend that if you need any surgery, including dental work, you should inform the practitioner that you're using gingko because it could cause increased bleeding.

### Zinc

*Zinc* is a mineral that is present in all organs, tissues, fluids and secretions of the body, and essential to human body function. Zinc is necessary for normal growth and development during pregnancy, childhood, and adolescence; immune system function; and wound healing. Changes in zinc absorption, excretion or increase on body requirement can result in zinc deficiency. This is particularly frequent in elderly people, vegetarians and alcoholics. Clinical manifestations include diarrhea, hair loss, muscle wasting, depression, irritability, and a rash involving the extremities, face, and perineum. Zinc deficiency has also been related to tinnitus.

Zinc has a protective effect on cochlear cells and can regulate nerve function activity related to tinnitus. Some preliminary trials suggest that administration of zinc could be beneficial to individuals with some kind of tinnitus and that it'll relieve tinnitus and maybe even prevent it. Zinc is generally well-tolerated. The most common side effects are poor digestion, abdominal pain and nausea.

## Vitamins

*Vitamins* are organic (natural) compounds required for essential reactions in the body. They're necessary for normal growth and development, maintenance of cells, tissues and organs. Many vitamins have been advocated to treat tinnitus, including b-carotene, vitamin C, vitamin E and vitamin B12. However, only vitamin B12 has been studied in a clinical trial for tinnitus.

## Vitamin B12 for Tinnitus

B12 is a vitamin essential for various functions of the body, including and neurologic functions. B12 deficiency is caused by dietary deficiency or a poor absorption by the body. Some people also appear to have an increased need. Vitamin B12 cannot be synthesized in the human body and must be supplied in the diet. The only dietary sources are animal products such as meat and dairy foods. Vitamin B12 deficiency might impair the vascular and nervous system of the auditory system and cause tinnitus. B12 might influence cochlear function and neural transmission and could potentially have an effect on tinnitus. Preliminary data has demonstrated improvement in some patients with tinnitus after receiving B12 supplements. Vitamin B12 supplements are usually well-tolerated. Side effects, which are often mild, include diarrhea, skin rashes and headaches.

## Teas

Many people with sleep problems choose herbal remedies for relief. For example, chamomile *tea* is known for its sedative properties. It's considered harmless for most people, but can cause allergic reactions in those who have plant or pollen allergies.

## Melatonin

*Melatonin* is a hormone produced by the pineal gland which is normally stimulated by darkness and inhibited by light. Melatonin helps to regulate sleep, which is a frequent complaint among tinnitus sufferers. Beneficial effects of melatonin improving night sleep have been reported, particularly in elderly patients with insomnia. Preliminary studies also suggest that melatonin decreases sleep problems in people with tinnitus.

## Valerian Root

*Valerian* is an herb. It is used to help people sleep, and might also help tinnitus sufferers with sleeping problems.

## Homeopathy

Proponents of *homeopathy* suggest it's based on the theory that it's possible to stimulate the body's defense mechanisms by giving small dosages of substances that would produce the illness if given in larger doses. The general thought is plausible, but the rationales for the homeopathic substances provided are vague, and the applications have no support in controlled studies. Proponents argue that the "remedies" are selected based on a total picture of the patient, the symptoms, emotional and mental states, lifestyle and other unspecified factors.   For more detailed information you might go to the following website: http://nccam.nih.gov/health/homeopathy/.

Some remedies which have been used for tinnitus include: calcarea carbonica, carbo vegetabilis, china, chininum sulphuricum, cimicifuga, coffee cruda, graphites, kali carbonicum, lycopodium, natrum salicylicum, and alicylicum acidum. No clinical trials of adequate methodology have demonstrated any efficacy of homeopathy to treat tinnitus.

## Reactions to Tinnitus

It is important to separate your tinnitus from your reactions to it. There are also treatments intended to treat your reactions, not your tinnitus. This is reasonable because as we've stated there's no widely accepted treatment that eliminates tinnitus or reduces its magnitude. Therefore, treating the reactions is a reasonable approach. The reactions people experience as a consequence of their tinnitus are typically problems with sleep, emotions, hearing and concentration (see also Chapters 4-6 and 8-9).

### Sleep Problems

Sleep problems are frequent complaints among tinnitus patients. Management of insomnia requires identification and resolution of stressful and precipitant causes. It's important to know that changes in your behavior and bedroom can be extremely helpful for sleep difficulties (see Chapter 8). Prolonged use of medications (that is, sleeping pills) can result in a dependency on the pills, which is undesirable. Medication and alternative treatments used to treat sleep problems are described next. Alternative treatments for sleep (teas, melatonin and valerian root) were previously described.

### Hypnotics

Drugs used specifically for improving sleeping are called *hypnotics*. The most prescribed medications are benzodiazepines and short-acting non-benzodiazepine hypnotics. These drugs should be reserved for acutely distressed patients and avoided among elderly. Because they create dependency, they should only be used for a short time. Medications should be withdrawn gradually and the patient should be aware of the possibility of sleep problems (*insomnia*). Drinking alcohol while taking sleep medications can intensify side-effects and should be avoided during the use of any sleep medication. These medications can only be used under medical prescription.

### Emotional Problems

Often tinnitus is associated with depression and anxiety. This is well-presented in Chapters 4-5 of this book so I won't delve into here.

## Depression

*Depression* is a state of intense sadness, melancholia or despair that has advanced to the point of being disruptive to an individual's social life and/or activities of daily living. Clinical depression is a clinical diagnosis and might be different from the everyday meaning of "being depressed." Medications that have been used to treat these symptoms are called *antidepressants*. The most used are the selective serotonin reuptake inhibitors, such as citalopram, fluoxetine, paroxetine and sertraline. Medications can help many people with severe depression. Counseling can also be very effective, even as an adjunct for depressed people taking medications.

## Anxiety

*Anxiety* is an unpleasant state associated with emotions that include apprehension, fear and worry. Some physical sensations might be present such as heart palpitations, nausea, chest pain, shortness of breath, or tension headache. The acute symptoms are most often controlled by anti-anxiety agents. The most commonly used are the benzodiazepines. However, they could induce dependency, so extended use should be carefully monitored by a physician.

## Attention, Concentration and Memory

Lack of attention, difficulties with concentration and loss of memory are often reported among tinnitus sufferers. These symptoms cause an impact on their quality of life, work and studying performances. Some recent findings from other areas of research have suggested that these difficulties might be linked related to specific chemicals (serotonin, noradrenaline and dopamine) that act in the brain, mainly in an area called the frontal cortex. There is some limited evidence that drugs that have an action on these chemicals might be able to improve these symptoms. Specific studies of these treatments among tinnitus patients have not been performed yet.

## Hearing Problems

Hearing loss is present in about 90% of tinnitus patients (see Chapters 2 and 7). For most types of hearing loss, there's no medication that can be helpful, but there are a few exceptions (see Chapter 11), including sudden hearing loss, Ménière's disease, noise and age-related hearing loss. The treatment requires a complete investigation and is directed at the cause. (See Chapters 7 and 10 for reviews of the causes of hearing loss and its treatments.) Generally, medications such as antibiotics, steroids, and drugs that act on blood circulation are used as treatments.

## Drugs that might Cause Tinnitus

There are many drugs used to treat other conditions that can result in tinnitus as a side effect. Of course, these drugs are prescribed with a purpose in mind, and stopping these medications should only be done with approval of your physician. Some medications can be substituted for another that might not produce tinnitus. Other prescribed medications might not have a reasonable substitute. It's also possible your physician will decide that it's possible to reduce the dosage of the medication which might eliminate the tinnitus. The benefits of taking the drug will have to be weighed against living with the tinnitus.

Although a large number of drugs present tinnitus as a side effect, not everyone will develop the symptom. Table 12-IV (next page) provides some examples of the more commonly prescribed drugs that can cause tinnitus. There are few drugs that can damage the ear or hearing and can cause tinnitus. They're called *ototoxic* and are mainly prescribed for severely ill patients. The risk to develop an ear disease has to be balanced with the effect that not taking the medication might have on your health. This group of drugs includes aminoglycoside antibiotics (for example, gentamicin) and cytotoxic drugs, used to treat cancer (for example, cisplatin).

## Conclusions

At this moment, there's no widely accepted medication or supplement that can cure tinnitus. However, there are several treatments that can alleviate or reduce some of the symptoms in some patients. There are many classes of prescription medications that have different mechanisms of action that might benefit some cases of tinnitus. Alternative treatments, including dietary supplements,

Table 12-IV: Medications that might cause tinnitus

<u>Analgesics/anti-inflammatories</u> to reduce pain and swelling:
aspirin, celecoxib, ibuprofen, piroxicam

<u>Antibiotics</u> taken to treat infections:
aminoglycosides (e.g. neomycin, streptomycin, gentamicin), clarithromycin, chloramphenicol, ciprofloxacin, erythromycin, tetracycline, vancomycin

<u>Antidepressants</u> used to treat depression:
amitriptyline, bupropion, doxepin, fluoxetine, imipramine, phenelzine, protriptyline, trazadone, venlafaxine

<u>Antihistamines</u> to prevent or reduce allergic reactions:
chlorpheniramine, loratadine

<u>Antimalarial meds</u> taken to prevent or to treat malaria:
chloroquinine, quinine

<u>Antivirals</u> taken to treat viral infections:
ganciclovir

<u>Anticonvulsants</u> taken to treat and prevent convulsions:
amitriptyline, carbamazepine

<u>Cardiac meds</u> taken to reduce high blood pressure:
amiloride, diltiazem, enalapril, furosemide, metoprolol, ramipril

<u>Chemoterapy drugs</u> taken to treat cancer:
bleomycin , cisplatin , mechlorethamine, methotrexate , vincristine

<u>Diuretics</u>:
bumetanide, ethacrynic acid, furosemide

have been used as tinnitus treatments. The fact that they are considered natural does <u>not</u> mean they're safe and don't cause adverse effects. Addressing specific reactions to tinnitus such as sleep, concentration, emotional and hearing problems is helpful and should be considered part of treatment. Some classes of medications might produce tinnitus as a side effect, and if this happens you should tell your physician as soon as it appears.

When you hear about a new cure for tinnitus, perhaps a newspaper article or story on the Internet, what should you do? Of course you want that pill to make it go away. Approach such cures cautiously. If there's a new study that has merit, it will be replicated, accepted and made known as a cure. If you seek a new treatment that has not been adequately studied, you might suffer serious side effects, waste your time and money, and make your tinnitus worse by giving it additional attention. Discuss new claims for a "cure" with your physician or audiologist before considering taking any treatment.

## Acknowledgments

I am grateful to Anne K. Gehringer for the valuable suggestions during the writing of this chapter.

# CHAPTER THIRTEEN

# Hyperacusis

## David M. Baguley BSc, MSc, MBA, PhD

*Director of Audiology, Addenbrooke's Hospital NHS Trust, Cambridge*

---

**Dr. Baguley** is a Consultant Clinical Scientist at Addenbrooke's Hospital, Cambridge. He studied psychology and then audiology at Manchester University and became Head of the Audiology Department at Addenbrooke's Hospital, Cambridge, in 1989. He has over 90 peer-review publications and a PhD from the University of Cambridge, and has peer-reviewed manuscripts for many learned journals including Brain. Dr. Baguley serves as Professional Advisor to the British Tinnitus Association and to the Royal National Institute for the Deaf Tinnitus Helpline.

---

## Introduction

Hearing is a remarkable sense, enabling us to hear an enormous range of sounds - from the delicate raindrop to the overwhelming jet engine. It's able to inform us quite precisely about the auditory environment by distinguishing very subtle differences in frequency, timing and intensity (see Chapter 7). One of the real puzzles is how our auditory system is able to code that enormously wide intensity range of sounds around us. We can hear a very quiet sound (a pin drop for example), but also sound that's very loud indeed (such as an emergency siren—though this sound would be uncomfortably loud). As with every other function of the human body, things can go wrong. For some people, sounds that would be moderately loud for most people are perceived as very loud and even annoying. As you know by now if you started reading from the start of this book, this annoyance is called *hyperacusis*. This chapter will explain this situation, the impact of this symptom, and what can be done about it.

At this stage it's important to make the distinction between the physical intensity (or level) of a sound, and the perceptual scale of loudness. In most circumstances, and for people whose hearing system is functioning well, there's a straightforward relationship between the two. As the intensity of a sound increases, it becomes louder. However, even for people with normal hearing, a sudden or unexpected sound can make them startle. And when people are anxious, such as when walking along an unfamiliar dark road, even a relatively soft sound can capture your attention and evoke fear. This indicates that the apparent loudness of sound is influenced by additional factors to the physical intensity.

## What is Hyperacusis?

One problem with understanding hyperacusis is that many different words are used, and this can be confusing for both patients and professionals. We'll use the word hyperacusis to mean the experience of moderately intense sounds, being perceived as very loud and annoying. Sometimes the word *phonophobia* is used when people develop a fear of sound. Although numerous other terms have been used, I believe that overall, "hyperacusis" is the best word to describe these symptoms.

In mild hyperacusis, moderately intense sounds (such as dishes banging together and the knife and fork clanging on the plate) are heard as loud. This can lead to stress, but most aspects of life can continue. In moderate cases you perceive many everyday sounds as very loud and annoying. You might even avoid some situations where you know there will be loud sounds, such as football games or concerts. You can become defensive and fearful, and might even think that the moderately intense sounds will harm you. At this point, many social activities are avoided, and family life can become a struggle.

In severe cases there is a very significant impact upon the individual and their family. Some people with hyperacusis constantly wear earplugs. Others notice this odd behavior. Not surprisingly the possibility of depression and chronic anxiety is significant, and these symptoms can add further to the hyperacusis. Here's an excerpt from the story of a lady with severe hyperacusis, who has now recovered:

"My partner and I were concerned about my apparent overreaction to moderately-intense noise. I was very anxious, wondering what was wrong with me, and wondering if it might be a brain tumor. Eventually, I couldn't bear to be in the kitchen (couldn't tolerate the noise of the kettle, boiler, microwave, and refrigerator), or use the vacuum cleaner, listen to music, TV, or play the piano. At its worst, I couldn't bear the noise of the hair dryer or even the sound of cutlery on the plates. Equally, I couldn't bear to be outside and sounds such as birds chirping, traffic (either close to or in the distance). Airplanes flying overhead were just so loud. Once I had a panic attack while listening to a very loud lawn mower. When we finally saw the audiologist, he allayed our fears by giving it a name (hyperacusis) and telling us that it was non-life threatening. However, hyperacusis took away many aspects of life because it's so limiting. I was unable to continue in my job as well as in my voluntary work and most of my social activities. I was even unable to travel either by car, bus, train or plane. Unable to go anywhere other than for quiet walks round the village. Unable to visit family or friends. Unable to work. It was difficult to talk to anyone on the phone, and I couldn't cook meals in the kitchen. It was like being a prisoner in my own home. Thankfully, my husband was able to arrange to work from home where he could do the cooking, as well as go with me wherever I went in case I had a panic attack."

Having severe hyperacusis can be very troubling indeed. You can become fearful, and isolated, trying to protect yourself from sound that you perceive to be intense and damaging. Work and family life can become affected as you become trapped in a vicious cycle of fear and increasing hyperacusis. As we'll see later though, recovery is possible.

It's interesting to consider how many people have hyperacusis. First, let us consider adults. A team of psychologists surveyed the people of Uppsala, Sweden, in two ways. The first was by a random postal survey, and the second was in a questionnaire on the website of a daily newspaper. Many hundreds of people replied, and in both groups just under 10% stated that they were bothered by sounds being very loud on that day. Some others have suggested that severe hyperacusis probably affects 1-2% of the adult population, but there's insufficient data yet to come to any firm conclusion. Even 1% of the population is a very large number of people!

Perhaps as many as 40% of people with troublesome tinnitus report hyperacusis. Also, the majority (maybe >90%) of people with severe hyperacusis report tinnitus. Many people with tinnitus and hyperacusis often note that the hyperacusis is more bothersome than the tinnitus. Although there is a relationship between tinnitus and hyperacusis (and with hearing loss), the precise nature of why they often coexist is not yet understood.

So much for adults—is it possible for children to have hyperacusis? The answer is Yes, but again we don't know how many. Fewer children than adults have hyperacusis, but when it's present, it can be very problematic for the child and the family.

## What causes Hyperacusis?

People with hyperacusis may understandably be very concerned about their situation, and the possibility that a sinister health condition may underlie it. This is rarely the case, however. The sensible course of action for someone with hyperacusis is to seek an informed clinical opinion from someone knowledgeable and interested in it. This might be from an *audiologist*, an *otolaryngologist*, or a *neurologist* (see Chapter 11).

Whilst not much is known about the causes of hyperacusis, a discussion with a knowledgeable clinician helps in deciding how to proceed with treatment even though it presently cannot be treated directly with surgery or medications. Sometimes an uninformed or dismissive opinion can do more harm than good.

In the consultation, the specialist will take a detailed history, and will determine if there are other health conditions present that may be associated with the hyperacusis (Table 13-I). In many cases there's no apparent relationship to another health condition. A review of medication will be undertaken, although associations between hyperacusis and specific medications are anecdotal at the present time.

Table 13-I: Health conditions that have been associated with hyperacusis (adapted from Baguley and Andersson, 2007)

| Peripheral | Central |
|---|---|
| Facial Palsy (Bell's Palsy) | Depression |
| Herpes Zoster Oticus | Post Traumatic Stress Disorder |
| (aka Ramsey-Hunt Syndrome) | Head injury |
| Stapedectomy | Obsessive-Compulsive Disorder |
|  | Lyme Disease |
|  | Migraine |

Particular attention will be paid to the onset of hyperacusis, and any life events or stresses that occurred around the same time. The presence of tinnitus, and other auditory symptoms, will be explored, alongside an examination of the ears and a hearing test (*audiogram*). Some audiologists will then go on to quantify the intensity of sound that is uncomfortable for the patient: this test is called a *Loudness Discomfort Level* test. Whilst there are a few variations in technique, you're typically asked to judge the loudness of a sound or to tell when a sound has become uncomfortably loud. There are also questionnaires available to quantify the impact of hyperacusis, and sometimes to determine the degree of anxiety or depression you also might be experiencing.

Particular health conditions sometimes associated with hyperacusis will also be considered. These can include head injury and facial palsy, though these are uncommon. People with migraine headaches sometimes complain of strong reactions to visual, olfactory and sound stimuli.

Very often the onset of hyperacusis is associated with exposure to intense sound, sometimes in circumstances where escape was impossible. This may have caused a permanent noise-induced hearing loss, which will be evident on the audiogram, but in some cases there may be no apparent physical damage to the inner ear (cochlea). As with tinnitus, there are likely many causes and mechanisms of hyperacusis. Hyperacusis is only a symptom.

When hearing loss is present, whether due to noise, aging or other factors, it's sometimes hard to understand why someone can find soft sounds hard to hear, but when the volume is increased, finds the sound hard to tolerate because it's so loud and annoying. In most forms of sensorineural hearing loss (see Chapter 7), quiet sounds are not heard below the threshold of hearing, but intense sounds are heard just as loud as they are by a normal hearing person. This is called *recruitment*.

Sometimes hyperacusis is associated with depression, or anxiety-related disorders (such as *post-traumatic stress disorder*). The link might be due to *neurotransmitter* issues (chemicals that brain cells use to communicate with each other; Chapter 3), but may also be due to the restriction of daily activities and limited sound exposure in the case of depression. Sometimes it's difficult to see which issue arose first, but it makes sense that if someone has both hyperacusis and depression, both symptoms deserve treatment.

In children, people have wondered about a link between hyperacusis and autism, and also with *Attention Deficit Hyperactivity Disorder* (ADHD). A child with hyperacusis should be examined by a *pediatrician* so that the range of possible childhood developmental diseases can be considered.

## The Mechanisms of Hyperacusis

In order to understand the mechanisms that may underlie hyperacusis I should first discuss how loudness of sound is usually perceived. Generally speaking, the intensity of a sound signal is proportional to the amount of nerve activity in the hearing system. In quiet surroundings, there's little nerve activity, and in intense noise there's a lot of nerve activity. The amount and spread of neural activity might be in error when hyperacusis is present. Also, the brain regulates some of its peripheral neural activity through the *efferent* neural system (see Chapter 3) by sending signals down from the brain to the *cochlea* (see Chapter 7). Some researchers believe that this efferent system might influence the loudness of sound, so it also might be at fault in hyperacusis. One further idea is that the neurotransmitter *serotonin* is involved coding sound and loudness. This is an interesting concept, since problems with serotonin are also involved in anxiety and depression, symptoms that often occur alongside hyperacusis.

Whenever an individual experiences an emotion, the *limbic system* is involved (see Chapter 3). There are direct links from all sensory systems to the limbic system, and these are especially strong between hearing and emotion. If people have an emotional reaction to the loudness of sounds, the limbic system must be involved. The association between hearing and emotion seems to be especially strong when fear and anxiety are concerned. The hearing system also has links to systems of reaction—the startle response to unexpected sudden sound is an indication of how quick and effective these links are. Interestingly, the links between hearing and reaction, and hearing and emotion are two-way, so that changes in emotion (such as anxiety) can increase our attention, as can increases in arousal (such as irritability).

All of these ideas lead us to the conclusion that looking at the ear alone in hyperacusis is not sufficient. In fact, recent work (Baguley and Andersson, 2007) has argued that in hyperacusis it's essential to consider a *biopsychosocial* perspective: that is to consider the biology (the ear), the psychology (emotions), and the social aspects (especially the family) of the situation. In this perspective each of these dimensions is seen as important and germane to understanding the situation. The biological dimension pertains to the ear and brain, considering the physiological mechanisms underpinning hyperacusis. The psychological aspects are also worthy of careful consideration, including both the emotions experienced by the individual, but also their cognitions (beliefs) regarding the situation. The social dimension is not only how the hyperacusis affects the person in their social environment, but also how the symptom is viewed in society in general. This latter aspect is particularly important for those individuals who believe themselves to be unable to function in environments (like supermarkets) without large earmuff hearing protection.

Another way to consider hyperacusis is to look at how it develops over time. In many individuals the onset is gradual and insidious. In others there are rapid changes from normal loudness perception to hyperacusis. In some cases there are obvious specific triggers (see examples listed in Table 13-II), but for others there seems to be no pattern at all. One way of looking at this has been to use something called a fear avoidance model (Figure 13-1) which suggests that the loudness, annoyance and fear of things becoming worse, all feed into each other and lead to a more severe hyperacusis. These three factors represented all interplay in the overall impact of hyperacusis.

Table 13-II. Some examples of *psychosocial* factors that can contribute to hyperacusis

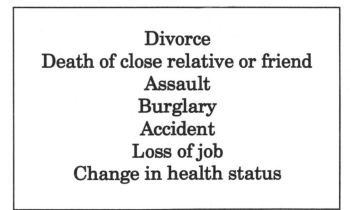

**Divorce**
**Death of close relative or friend**
**Assault**
**Burglary**
**Accident**
**Loss of job**
**Change in health status**

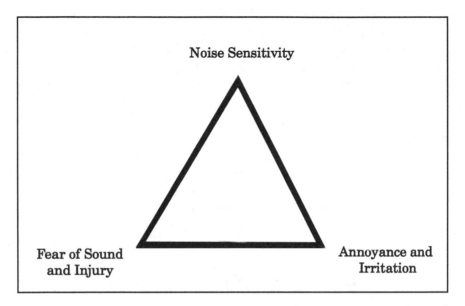

Figure 13-1: Three component model of hyperacusis (adapted from Baguley and Andersson, 2007)

In order to understand how a person can develop hyperacusis, and how they can recover, we should consider how the brain can change and adapt. This ability is referred to as *plasticity* and underpins human learning—like learning a new language. Craig Formby, PhD, and his colleagues at the University of Maryland had normal hearing volunteers (with no hyperacusis) wear earplugs 23 hours per day. After two weeks, they took their earplugs off and had them rate the loudness of sounds using loudness scaling tests. These normal listeners judged moderately loud sounds as very loud! Another group of normal hearing volunteers wore noise generators all day long. After two weeks, they took off the noise generators. These normal listeners judged loud sounds as only moderately loud! These ingenious experiments shows mechanisms of brain plasticity in the hearing system at work, and has major implications for strategies to recover from hyperacusis (next section).

### What Therapies are Available?

Some good news is that therapies are emerging for hyperacusis. As in tinnitus, the components of therapy include counseling and sound therapy. Because hyperacusis may be accompanied by hearing loss, hearing aids also play a role. Since many people with severe hyperacusis use hearing protection, it'll be important to discuss this. Many relaxation procedures, formal and informal, can also be helpful for those with hyperacusis. Self help is a major benefit in hyperacusis, and ways of getting started with this are considered in the next section.

## Counseling

Professionals who provide counseling for hyperacusis often separate the process into two components. First is providing information about hearing, hearing loss, and hyperacusis. The chapters in this book are designed to do just that. Whatever the disorder, most people appreciate a deeper understanding of possible causes, mechanisms and treatments, and hyperacusis is no exception. Often it's desirable to provide this information to all those affected by the hyperacusis, and in particular the spouse or partner.

A second component of the counseling involves understanding and changing your reactions to your hyperacusis. Like tinnitus, there probably are many different forms of hyperacusis. Some people with hyperacusis, particularly the more severe forms when distress reactions of annoyance and fear are present, develop unrealistic thoughts and expectations about the effects of sound in their environment. It's important to understand your beliefs and thoughts about sound intensities, and their potential (or lack thereof) to harm your hearing. It's also helpful to review how you react to sound, and consider if these are really appropriate reactions or not.

## Sound Therapy

The important experiment by Dr. Craig Formby, as previously described, shows that the use of noise can help the hearing system adjust to loud environmental sounds. This is useful evidence, and supports the use of sound therapy in hyperacusis. I will describe two main approaches.

When someone is uncommonly afraid of spiders, a useful approach is incremental gradual exposures. This is sometimes called *successive approximations.* This might begin by viewing a picture of a spider, then a plastic model of a spider, and finally an encounter with a real spider. One form of sound therapy for hyperacusis also involves this desensitization procedure. This was originally proposed by Jack Vernon, PhD. In this technique, broadband noise is initially introduced at a soft level and then gradually increased over some weeks. There might be specific listening times, such as the hour before bed, or the exposure to sound could be all the waking day. The next week the sound level would be increased slightly, and then again the next week, and the next, and so on. The idea is to "desensitize" the hearing system gradually. The sound-producing device can be wearable or non-wearable. The options are the same as for tinnitus treatments, and are defined in detail in Chapter 10. Another slightly different sound therapy approach is to introduce noise at a fixed low level. This level is audible, but well below that which causes discomfort and remains at that level allowing the hearing system to reset (or recalibrate) itself to that sound.

Both these approaches have their advocates, and at the present time there's little rigorous scientific evidence to help choose between them. Both approaches are reasonable, and unlikely to do harm, so at the present time it's a matter of preference.

In both strategies, a considerable amount of time, and consistent use of the sound therapy, is required—but what's also common to both is the hope that eventually the hearing system will recover from its abnormal coding of intensity and the use of sound therapy will no longer be required.

### Relaxation

We all have to deal with stress in our lives, and finding effective ways to relax is good for all of us. Of course hyperacusis would cause agitation, arousal and distress for any of us. One thing you can do for yourself is to follow good practices to keep the stress in your life tolerable, and to follow some behaviors that can help keep you relaxed. Although we all relax in different ways, these might include:

- exercising
- taking time for yourself
- listening to soft music
- performing an enjoying relaxing hobby

Other people with hyperacusis seem to benefit more from more formal relaxation approaches. These include: the use of yoga, Pilates techniques and swimming.

The use of *progressive muscle relaxation* therapy can be particularly helpful. This technique uses a mixture of physical tensing/relaxing techniques, breathing exercises and mental imagery to reduce agitation and arousal (see also Chapters 5 and 8-9). Over time and with practice, the effect becomes instinctive. This technique can be learned from self-help books, videos, television shows or from a professional trained in the technique (usually with better results).

## Hearing Aids

Some people with hyperacusis also have hearing loss, and will likely benefit from hearing aids. Hearing aids amplify sound, and this is exactly the opposite of what most people with hyperacusis want. Therefore, hearing aid fitting in someone with hyperacusis should be undertaken with great care.

First, it's important to realize that all hearing aids have the ability to limit their maximum output. This is performed using output *compression limiting* or in older analog devices, *peak clipping,* although the latter is rarely used anymore. The aid is set such that it will allow only a defined maximum output, no matter what the level of the incoming sound. An audiologist will usually check this by creating brief intense sounds (like vigorous hand clapping) to ensure that this maximum output limiting is not exceeded.

In someone with hyperacusis, the maximum output of a hearing aid can be set at a very low level. It should be appreciated that this limits the dynamic range of speech that can be presented through the hearing aid. This represents a trade-off. In time, as confidence builds and as your hearing adapts to amplification, the maximum output of the hearing aid can be carefully and slowly increased. This often takes several visits and reprogramming sessions. Thus, eventually the dynamic range of hearing can be gradually increased and optimized while at the same time external sounds should not be perceived as too loud.

## Hearing Protection

All audiologists agree that hearing protection should always be used when there's a chance that intense sounds could damage the auditory system. This is true for everyone. However, it's quite common for people with hyperacusis to overprotect themselves from everyday sounds by using earplugs or other forms of hearing protection for moderately intense sounds when there's really no chance of harming their hearing. In such a situation the earplug use is driven by fear as much as by any real risk.

Several clinicians have suggested that in hyperacusis the use of hearing protection to reduce exposure to moderately intense sounds can make hyperacusis significantly worse. Because the sound sent up to the brain is reduced, the brain must somehow recalibrate itself and perhaps in effect turns up the volume to achieve normal levels of activity. Therefore, the overuse of hearing protection for people with hyperacusis carries considerable risk of making things worse.

To summarize these thoughts, it's generally agreed that someone with hyperacusis should: use hearing protection when background sounds are intense enough, but refrain from using hearing protection when there's no threat of hearing damage because the background sounds are not potentially damaging.

There is an intermediate step. The use of hearing protection can start with events that are expected (or feared) to have high intensity sound (such as use when shopping or when out on the street for fear of unexpected sounds). Eventually, gradual exposure without hearing protection at these events is needed. If absolutely necessary - for instance to be able to attend a wedding or a funeral - then hearing protection can be justified, but for that event only. For such events the use of inexpensive musician's earplugs can be helpful. They're not as effective at limiting noise exposure as other earplugs, but they *attenuate* noise equally across the frequency range, so that speech is easier to understand (and music is clearer). During therapy, many clinicians will work with patients to reduce use of hearing protection over time.

## How can I Help Myself?

There are several straightforward things that people with hyperacusis can do to help themselves. The first is to learn about, and to understand the situation. The effect of clear and accurate information can be dramatic and should not be underestimated. Similarly, the devastating effect of pessimistic information can be catastrophic, and care should be taken in which information to read. This chapter is a start, and the realistic but cautiously optimistic tone is intended to be encouraging. Common sense and caution is advised when reading on the Internet. People who are recovering may not be motivated to post on message boards, leaving the way clear for the minority who are trapped in severe hyperacusis. Whilst genuine and well-motivated, many such people do not realize the devastation their posts can cause. You are on safer ground with the moderated boards provided by the Hyperacusis Network* which organization is a source of much valuable information and resources.

Formal sound therapy for hyperacusis can also be helpful. There are ways of undertaking this on an informal basis. Sources of helpful sound that can be accessed informally and relatively inexpensively include the variety of table top music and environmental sound generators which are available. These make sounds like rain and ocean waves, and can be used quietly to increase one's acceptance and interpretation of intense sound (see Chapter 10).

The potential benefit of hearing aids when the maximum output is appropriately set for people with hearing loss and hyperacusis has already been discussed. Whilst some audiologists may not have extensive experience with hyperacusis, they will know their hearing aid science, and with some discussion will be able to initially set the maximum output to a lower level, and then increase the maximum output in a gradual, safe and incremental manner.

As discussed earlier, the use of hearing protection presents a real risk for people with hyperacusis. The use of earplugs should be minimized when harmful sound is not present, and individuals are encouraged to wean themselves off their use. Speak to friends and family about the sound environment you are concerned about. Try to determine if there's a real risk of noise injury and the extent to which fear and anxiety are involved in your hearing protection use.

Informal strategies for relaxation have been discussed, and are commonsense for all of us (including audiologists!). Care should be taken to continue use of such strategies, even when recovery from hyperacusis is underway, as they may have an important role in relapse prevention.

*The Hyperacusis Network (http://www.hyperacusis.net/) aims to share information about hyperacusis coordinated by laypersons. Information is given about various tactics people have used, and a message board provides discussion about the topic.

Having formal therapy for hyperacusis is not the only option. The elements of information, sound therapy and relaxation therapy are found throughout this book, and are summarized in Table 13-III.

Table 13-III: Beginner's guide to hyperacusis self-help

> 1. **Get informed! (this chapter is a start)**
> 2. **Get an educated clinical opinion from a well-informed professional**
> 3. **Adopt relaxation strategies**
> 4. **Wean yourself off hearing protection except when exposed to intense sound**
> 5. **Use sound therapy (formal or informal)**

Even after recovery from hyperacusis through formal therapy, you'll have to continue taking good care of yourself. Below are some reflections from one of our patients who is recovering from severe hyperacusis:

"An example of working around the hyperacusis is by doing some of the things that I like, such as having a coffee in town. Most cafés are noisy especially on Saturdays, but we get round the problem by going into town very early, to a bookshop where there are some quiet alcoves with benches and comfy chairs. My husband gets the coffees from a nearby café and we sit in peace and quiet reading and enjoying the coffee break.

"There's plenty of evidence for improvement in the hyperacusis. For example, in late December I noticed a man mowing his lawn. The first thought was that it was very odd for anyone to be mowing their lawn in the middle of winter. Only later did it dawn on me that I hadn't noticed the drone of the lawnmower and that this sound was no longer uncomfortable or distressing.

"In the last two years, the hyperacusis has improved slowly but overall, tremendously. I still avoid going to places where I'm not in control of the sound environment, for example, certain working environments, shops with very loud intrusive music, concerts, cinema and dances. We changed the car for a much quieter one and I can now travel (and drive) at 70 mph, enabling me to visit family and friends again, as well as go on holiday.

"As my confidence increased, I was able to travel by train again (to France on the Euro Tunnel), by ferry and sea-cat. For some time now I have been able to accept all normal household noises including the food processor and the vacuum cleaner (a noisy brute!) "

## A Future for Hyperacusis

In the last 10 years, there has been a lot of interest in researching and treating hyperacusis. Despite this, a concern among people with hyperacusis is that no one's interested and that no research is being undertaken. Whilst there is indeed widespread ignorance about or indifference to the symptom among many in the healthcare community, it's also the case that there's a growing body of clinicians and hearing researchers that are interested, and that are undertaking basic and clinical research. Nearly all of the remarks made in Chapter 14 on the American Tinnitus Association's Roadmap to the Cure are applicable also to hyperacusis.

There are many new research themes involving hyperacusis. The role of the auditory efferent system is being investigated, and the possibility that this may underlie hyperacusis. The biochemical basis of hyperacusis is also being considered, with the potential prospect that this may be influenced by prescribed drugs being of great importance. There are hearing scientists researching how loudness is coded within the hearing portions of the brain, and how this changes with hearing loss. Finally, the use of sound therapy for hyperacusis is being researched, with particular emphasis upon optimizing the sound.

Without a crystal ball it's not possible to tell when all this work will bear fruit. What is a great encouragement, however, is the fact that the hearing science community is taking hyperacusis seriously, and is determined to improve therapy for individuals whose lives are affected by it.

## Summary

Hyperacusis can be a life-altering symptom for affected individuals and their families. In this chapter, the following points have been made:

- hyperacusis is the abnormal perception of loudness, and is sometimes accompanied by annoyance and fear;
- it's not known how common it is, but it's often accompanied by hearing loss and tinnitus;
- the mechanism of hyperacusis is not known, but likely includes the central auditory pathways including the brain;
- there's no accepted cure for hyperacusis at this time;
- therapy is available, and include counseling and sound therapy (further clinical trials are needed to document their success);
- relaxation exercises should be helpful for most people with hyperacusis;
- people with hyperacusis and hearing loss can wear hearing aids if the maximum output of the aid is limited;
- hearing protection should be used in the presence of potentially damaging noise, but is likely counterproductive for someone with hyperacusis in the presence of moderately intense sounds;
- research is underway and there's hope for cures and refined treatments in the future.

In writing this chapter it has been my hope that you would use this information to get to better manage your hyperacusis. Whilst a magic cure presently eludes us, there are well-established strategies for reducing hyperacusis that are readily available. There are things you can and should do, and I hope they bring you great benefit.

### Acknowledgements

This chapter was written while David was a Raine Visiting Professor at the Ear Science Institute, University of Western Australia. The Raine Foundation, Phonak Pty and the British Tinnitus Association are thanked for their support. Grateful thanks are given to the anonymous patient whose account is used in this chapter.

### Reference

Baguley DM, Andersson G (2007) Hyperacusis: Diagnosis, Mechanisms and Therapy. San Diego: Plural Publishers.

## Further Reading

Formby, C., Sherlock, L. P., & Gold, S. L. (2003). Adaptive plasticity of loudness induced by chronic attenuation and enhancement of the acoustic background. *Journal of the Acoustical Society of America,* 114, 55-58.

# CHAPTER FOURTEEN

# The American Tinnitus Association and The Roadmap to a Cure

## James A. Kaltenbach, PhD
*Wayne State University School of Medicine, Detroit, MI*

## David P. Fagerlie, MSW
*Chief Executive Officer, the American Tinnitus Association, Portland, OR*

**Dr. Kaltenbach** is Professor of Otolaryngology at Wayne State University (WSU) School of Medicine. He obtained his PhD in Biology at the University of Pennsylvania in 1984, then completed a three-year postdoctoral fellowship in physiology, also at the University of Pennsylvania. He joined the Department of Audiology at WSU in 1987 where he taught courses in auditory anatomy and physiology, psychoacoustics, and clinical instrumentation. In 1995, he joined the Department of Otolaryngology. His research has been supported by federal, corporate and private agencies for over 25 years and focuses on the neurobiological basis of hearing disorders, including noise-induced hearing loss, ototoxicity and tinnitus.

**David Fagerlie** received his MSW in administration and planning from the School of Social Work at the University of Washington. He also studied the marketing of not-for-profit organizations at the School of Business and established a marketing program for a large home healthcare agency. He has been Chief Executive Officer for the American Tinnitus Association since 2006. Before joining ATA, he had a Seattle, Washington-based consulting practice providing organizational change and human resource services. He has also served as assistant vice president for alumni affairs at the University of Washington in Seattle and worked in the United Way field in three states. His early career was in the aging and healthcare field.

There are millions of people with tinnitus all around the world. You are not alone! Many with tinnitus have formed self-help groups with regular meetings. The intent is to share information and provide support. The first organization of its kind, the American Tinnitus Association, was established to provide information and fund research.

## In the Beginning - the Power of the Pen

The first organization in the world formed to address tinnitus was the American Tinnitus Association founded in 1971 by Charles Unice, MD. Dr. Unice, a tinnitus sufferer, sought to create an organization that would raise money to fund research for a cure. He soon called Jack Vernon, PhD, the one tinnitus researcher in the world at the time. Dr. Vernon explained he could not offer Unice treatment for tinnitus as none existed. Even so, three days later Unice showed up at Vernon's office in Portland. During a walk that afternoon while standing near a water fountain in downtown Portland, Unice discovered he could not hear his tinnitus. It was a "Eureka!" moment for Vernon who understood immediately what had happened. The sound of the flowing water masked Unice's tinnitus, providing him with welcome relief. "Obviously, we can't park Unice next to the fountain for the rest of his life," Vernon thought. "But we might be able to replicate the fountain's sound in some sort of wearable device." That's how Vernon developed wearable masking devices (see Chapter 10). Jack Vernon became a co-founder of the American Tinnitus Association and the driving force behind funding tinnitus research at a time when no other support existed.

Gloria Reich, PhD joined the American Tinnitus Association in 1975 and later became its first Executive Director. She and Vernon developed a tinnitus training course for healthcare professionals and brought it to communities throughout the country. Although resources were limited, in 1980, American Tinnitus Association awarded its first research grant in the amount of $12,000.

Though formed to be a fundraising machine to support research, in looking back, one could conclude that the major contribution American Tinnitus Association made in its first decade was as source of comfort for those who were suffering. So little was known. No established protocols for treatment or therapeutic devices existed. Tinnitus sufferers and their loved ones feared that this condition was a sign the affected person was going crazy. American Tinnitus Association became an association of individuals - the afflicted, their families, and informed healthcare professionals - sharing information, support and encouragement.

In 1978, the syndicated newspaper publication <u>Parade</u> ran an article on tinnitus and the American Tinnitus Association efforts to provide information to the public. Over 100,000 pieces of mail, many with donations, arrived at the American Tinnitus Association door over the next few weeks. It took three full months for the nascent staff to respond to the overflow of mail. In 1983, the syndicated newspaper column "Dear Abby" mentioned tinnitus and referenced American Tinnitus Association. The office received another 20,000 letters. Mentions in "Dear Abby" and "Ann Landers" columns in 1986 produced another 130,000 letters. Contributions from so much public attention were the seed capital that moved the association forward. American Tinnitus Association's reputation as the center of tinnitus information expanded throughout the USA and into other countries.

Today, American Tinnitus Association remains the largest association of individual contributors making grants for tinnitus research. Similar associations are now present in other countries, mostly to provide support for those with tinnitus (see Table 10-I at end of this chapter).

Also today, tinnitus may very well be the "malady" of the 21st century. Early on, opportunities for growth were not as straightforward as they are today. These days tinnitus is being openly discussed and media organizations regularly report about it. American Tinnitus Association has increased its momentum toward educating community and government leaders and inspiring greater philanthropy. American Tinnitus Association has assumed a leadership role to rid the world of a scourge that is silent and unseen to those unaffected but shreds quality of life for a rapidly increasing number of adults, youth, and children. We need American Tinnitus Association and organizations like it more than ever before.

American Tinnitus Association was established specifically to raise money for tinnitus research. Before 1925 only nineteen scientific papers about tinnitus had been published. Progress was slow. In the ten-year period between 1955 and 1964, fifty-two reports were published. From 1965 to 1974 the number increased dramatically to 472 published works on tinnitus. When the American Tinnitus Association made its first grant in 1980, it was the first by any organization given specifically for the study of tinnitus.

In the late 1990s, it became clear that a general plan might be needed to help find the cure. The American Tinnitus Association again took a leadership role by recognizing that many scientists and clinicians were needed from different disciplines, and so a roadmap to a cure would be helpful.

## The American Tinnitus Association Roadmap to a Cure

In 2005, American Tinnitus Association unveiled its Roadmap to a Cure which was developed by members of its Scientific Advisory Committee (Figure 14-1). The backbone of the roadmap is the sequence of 4 goals shown in the left column. The paths to the right of each goal show the research steps needed to complete these goals. Cures for tinnitus will be realized when research has achieved the objectives set forth in each of the 4 paths.

The roadmap is important because it identifies what we now know, and what we need to know, in order to make progress toward a cure. The roadmap prioritizes areas of study, highlights opportunities, and reveals knowledge gaps. It can accelerate the speed of research, and help shorten the path between research and finding a cure. In the process, research accomplishments lead to improved treatments. The roadmap is also helpful for people with tinnitus to understand research needs, in tracking research progress, and to philanthropists in helping them to better target their support.

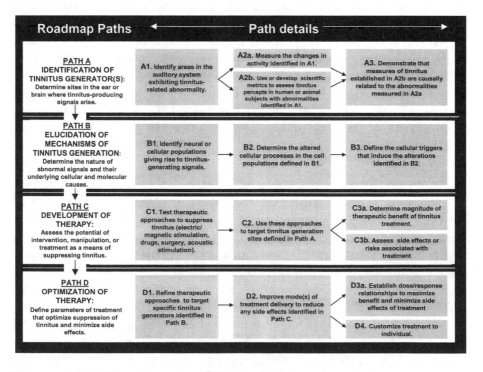

Figure 14-1: The American Tinnitus Association's Roadmap to a Cure developed by the Scientific Advisory Committee

## Introduction

The discovery of a cure for a disease or other health disorder might be thought of as a breakthrough moment in research resulting in a long sought-after magic bullet that works for most people. We share the dream that someday such a panacea will be found that works for tinnitus in the same way that, say, Motrin works for headaches. But how long will it take? Based on past experience, it seems that a breakthrough "cure" is most likely to occur if we have a strategy that allows research to move progressively by building a framework of knowledge.

But how should research proceed to find such a cure? What directions are best? There are many possible ways to seek a cure. Examples include clinical testing of drugs, maskers, or other treatment approaches that have been found to be helpful for some people. But we would be in a better position to develop treatment if we knew which mechanisms in the brain or ear contributed to the production of tinnitus (see Chapters 3 and 7). There are many ways to do this as well: should we use brain imaging (see Chapter 11) to see in which areas of the brain the problem lies? Or should we go more basic, and attempt to induce tinnitus in animals that help pin down the defects that underlie tinnitus? Clearly, there are numerous approaches to advance our understanding of tinnitus. But how do all these approaches come together to move us closer to that "cure" we seek? What will put the field of tinnitus research into exponential motion?

The roadmap to a cure was developed by the American Tinnitus Association, not so much with the intention of plotting a single path to a cure, but rather to illustrate how the various approaches toward seeking a cure can be tied together. A crossword puzzle provides clues for each word, and the numbers in the grid show how the words intersect with each other. In the same way, the roadmap provides the clues that need to be pursued by the scientific community, and shows how the knowledge gained will tie together. The roadmap has other benefits along the way, for in understanding how knowledge from all the different types of studies tie together, we'll be able to measure progress, identify areas of research that need more emphasis, and define target areas for research funding. All these benefits will help motivate researchers to seek better means of treating tinnitus.

The roadmap in its present form consists of four paths, each of which is defined by a general goal and consists of several specific strategies or steps toward achievement of that goal. The goal of Path A is to identify the sites and abnormalities giving rise to tinnitus signals. In other words, Path A helps define <u>where</u> in the ear or brain tinnitus is located. Path B is oriented toward what researchers refer to as the mechanisms of tinnitus generation, or <u>how</u> the brain produces the tinnitus sound The aim of Path C is to develop effective treatments for tinnitus, and that of Path D is to optimize those treatments for each individual. Below is a more detailed explanation of the steps needed to accomplish these goals. As we'll see, these paths are not independent but rather intersect with each other like a crossword puzzle.

## Path A: Identifying the Tinnitus Generators

The goal of Path A research is to define the generators of tinnitus. This goal requires completion of the following three steps.

**Step 1.** This is concerned with identifying areas in the *auditory system* exhibiting tinnitus-related abnormalities. This step identifies the parts of the auditory system that act differently in people with tinnitus. The challenge here is to define the nature of the abnormalities associated with tinnitus and determine where they occur. Since the nervous system uses electrical signals to communicate information, changes in these signals or in the way the information is communicated are considered abnormalities (see Chapter 3). Such changes would likely be found in the auditory portion of the nervous system (referred to globally as the auditory system), although areas outside the auditory system also need to be considered as sources of tinnitus signals. Techniques for demonstrating these alterations include electrophysiological recording techniques (see Chapter 11) from areas or groups of nerve cells (*neurons*) or from single neurons.

There are also several techniques available for visualizing or imaging the brains of subjects with tinnitus (see Chapter 11). Such methods include positron emission tomography (PET); single photon emission computed tomography (SPECT); functional magnetic resonance imaging (fMRI); magnetoencephalography (MEG); near infrared spectoscopic imaging (NIRSI); and multichannel electroencephalography (EEG). Both electrophysiological recordings and imaging techniques can be carried out in human subjects or in animals treated with substances that might induce tinnitus (such as aspirin). As the range of techniques expands and the imaging technologies become more sensitive and sophisticated, they can be expected to pinpoint the sources of tinnitus producing abnormalities with more and more precision.

**Step 2.** This path focuses on developing measures of the abnormalities identified in Step 1 and measures of tinnitus. Systematic measurements are key to being able to demonstrate a relationship between an abnormality and tinnitus. One needs measures that show the magnitude of the abnormality and how the magnitude varies in a given auditory structure to understand the kind of sound perception it's likely to produce. Similarly, measures of tinnitus are essential to understand what people hear and how it relates to the activity changes in the auditory system. Human studies can show whether certain abnormalities are found only in certain subgroups of subjects with specific forms of tinnitus.

**Step 3.** This addresses the question of which of the abnormalities identified in Steps 1 and 2 actually cause tinnitus. This is a much more demanding step because several types of abnormalities have been identified in animals (to be discussed later in this chapter) and humans with tinnitus and the future may reveal many more. It must be determined which of these abnormalities is the actual cause of tinnitus and which is a just background accompaniment. This is the job of separating the wheat from the chaff. The types of questions that need answers are: Does the abnormality occur only when tinnitus is present but not when it is absent? Since tinnitus is often accompanied by hearing loss, is the abnormality more related to tinnitus than hearing loss? Does the suspected abnormality increase in degree with increasing severity of tinnitus? And does reduction of the abnormality results in the reduction of tinnitus?

## Path B: Elucidation of Tinnitus Mechanisms

The goal of Path B research is to understand the mechanisms underlying tinnitus. This path has three steps. Step 1 is to identify the population of cells that are generating the abnormality identified in Path A. Step 2 is to define the chemical and anatomical defects in these cells which leads them to produce their abnormal activity. Step 3 is to figure out what causes these defects.

**Step 1.** This identifies the population of cells that are generating the abnormal activity which is a subtle issue that can be compared to a mechanic trying to diagnose the cause of an obnoxious rattling noise coming from the back end of a car. The mechanic might already know that the noise is coming from the wheel. But is it a strut? Is it a bushing? Or is it the hubcap? Knowing what the specific component is in the larger assembly of the wheel is key to being able to fix the problem. In the case of the tinnitus generator, each structure of the nervous system, whether a nerve, a nucleus, such as the dorsal cochlear nucleus, or a cortical area, such as the auditory cortex, consists of thousands of cells (see Chapter 3). These cells are classified into several different categories based on their shapes, sizes, connections with other neurons and their physiological properties. We may already know from Path A research what general structures produce the tinnitus signals (*cochlear nucleus, inferior colliculus* or *auditory cortex*), but further research is needed to find out what cell types are generating the abnormal firing pattern. This may be necessary because blocking the activity of the wrong cell population could cause a worsening of tinnitus.

**Step 2.** Once the abnormal cell type is identified, there's need to identify the chemical and anatomical defects in those cells that cause their electrical activity to change. This is a multi-layered problem. At one level, we need to know what chemical changes in the cell cause the defect. For example, if tinnitus is caused by hyperactivity of neurons, then we must find out what's causing neurons to be hyperactive. Is it because they're being overdriven by other excitatory neurons? Or are they overactive because there has been anatomical damage to other neurons that normally inhibit them? Is the defect caused by alterations in the cell's genetic code? That is, are some genes mutated or switched on when they should be off; or vice versa?

**Step 3.** The last step of Path B is to define the triggers that induce the defects in the abnormal cell populations. This aim is necessary because, although it may be clear which cell populations are firing abnormally and what the underlying defect is, our ability to correct the defect may benefit from knowing what caused the defect to develop in the first place. For example, we might want to know why noise exposure causes loss of neurons or synapses (the connections between neurons) that produce inhibitory effects on other neurons (see Chapter 3). Excessive noise exposure or loss of hearing with age causes deficiencies in the *neurotransmitters* that normally function to keep activity in certain cells quiet. These are referred to as inhibitory neurotransmitters. If it's found that noise-induced tinnitus is caused by a loss of inhibitory neurotransmitter function, what changes trigger the loss of that function? Is it hearing loss? Or is it destruction of outer hair cells in the inner ear (see Chapter 7)? How important is damage to the auditory nerve? We know that excessive stimulation of the ear by sound can cause chemical damage to auditory nerve or brain cells. How important is this type of change? Why do some triggers cause temporary tinnitus while others cause a more chronic form of tinnitus? More work is needed to determine which of these potential triggers is most important.

### Path C: Development of Therapy

The goal of Path C is to find therapeutic approaches that will bring relief to tinnitus patients. The steps in this path might be thought of as a gradual progression from the general to the more specific. How specific depends on the extent to which they use knowledge obtained from Paths A and B. This is explained more clearly as follows:

**Step 1.** The first step is to test approaches that have the potential to become useful anti-tinnitus therapies. In this initial step, the approaches are usually expected to be relatively primitive and make only preliminary attempts to build on knowledge produced by research in Paths A and B. Many studies in this step might test a new type of treatment in a small number of patients. Some may use animal models developed in Path A research to determine whether one of the treatment modalities has a significant anti-tinnitus effect. Because of their preliminary nature, approaches tested in this step are expected to have only a partial benefit or bring relief to only a few patients.

**Steps 2 and 3.** These steps strive to improve treatment approaches developed in Step 1. They're guided significantly by knowledge gained from research in Path A. Research in Step 2 might seek to further develop treatment methods that target the tinnitus generators identified in Path A. For example, a Step 2 study might build on the knowledge that tinnitus-related hyperactivity originates in different parts of the brainstem, such as the dorsal cochlear nucleus or the inferior colliculus (see Chapter 3). Alternatively, Step 2 research could target areas that are involved in the emotional response to tinnitus, a discovery made during Path A research. Because Step 2 research directly targets one or more of the tinnitus generator sites or the areas giving rise to the emotional disturbances caused by tinnitus, the effects of treatment are expected to be stronger and the benefit greater. It's also expected that this direct approach would provide tinnitus suppression at lower doses of treatment and thus fewer side effects would be likely. This would be demonstrated by careful measurements of the degree of tinnitus suppression, the percentage of subjects showing benefit and the severity of side effects.

## Path D: Optimization of Therapy

Path D is oriented toward the optimization of treatments developed in Path C. It's not unlikely that Path C research would lead to treatments that work for a significant percentage, maybe even a large majority of subjects with tinnitus. But the treatments achieved in Path C would be less than optimal. A treatment that reduces tinnitus may cause or worsen hearing loss, may work well in a limited percentage of patients, or the tinnitus may still be present even if it's greatly reduced or becomes less disturbing.

**Step 1.** The first step in this path builds on knowledge obtained in Path B which defined both the population of cells within the tinnitus generating sites that are firing abnormally, and the defect in those cells leading to that abnormality. For example, research in this step might be aimed at refining the therapy tested in Path C by reducing the activity of the abnormal nerve cell populations. This might be achieved by chemically activating a subclass of inhibitory receptors that is found only on cells that are hyperactive. Alternatively, one might test the effect of electrically or acoustically activating a pathway that provides inhibitory input to the hyperactive cells.

**Steps 2 and 3.** Research in the second step of Path D seeks to improve modes of treatment delivery to reduce any side effects identified in Path C. Side effects could include auditory symptoms, such as hearing loss or hyperacusis (see Chapter 13) or any other hearing deficit. They could also include non-auditory symptoms, such as drowsiness, nausea, sleeplessness, changes in heart rate, or decline in psychological well-being. Improvement in treatment delivery mode will vary for each type of therapy. One example of how treatment delivery modes can be improved is seen in pain treatment using morphine. The dose of this drug required to achieve pain reduction is lower and the severity and incidence of side effects greatly diminished by administering the drug intrathecally (that is, directly into the cerebrospinal fluid via a spinal implant) than through an intravenous line (a tube into a blood vessel) or skin patch. Electrical suppression of tinnitus symptoms might be greatly improved with fewer side effects with multiple sites of stimulation than with a single site, or by optimizing the time and frequency at which the stimulation is delivered. It may be possible to achieve greater reductions of tinnitus with fewer side effects by administering more than one drug to eliminate abnormal electrical activity at many levels of the auditory system. Ultimately, these improvements will involve fine tuning of treatments already available. Fine tuning will be possible only through measuring how different patients respond to different treatments. There may be need to customize treatment for each individual. That is, a dose of drug or a combination of treatments may have to be varied for each individual to determine the optimal conditions of treatment. Individualized treatment will likely be necessitated by the fact that tinnitus has many different causes and characteristics. Also, even when the characteristics and causes are similar, patients differ widely in how their lives are affected by their tinnitus.

## Progress in the Roadmap

### Path A Progress

**Step 1.** Important progress toward the goal of identifying tinnitus-related abnormalities in the nervous system has been made over the past decade: 1) The discovery that tinnitus-inducing agents alter neural activity in several ways. First, neurons in the auditory system do become hyperactive in certain structures. This means that their resting (spontaneous) activity increases as though they were responding to sound, even though no sound is present (see Chapter 3). Also, in some structures, neurons become more likely to fire at the same time (to be more synchronized) and/or they become more likely to fire in bursts rather than at regularly spaced intervals. 2) It's becoming increasingly apparent that some forms of tinnitus originate in the ear or auditory nerve. Salicylate, the active ingredient in aspirin (a well-known inducer of tinnitus) causes hyperactivity to occur in the auditory nerve. This hyperactivity appears to start in the inner ear. Other forms of tinnitus appear to involve hyperactivity that starts in the brain. There's now evidence that the hyperactivity induced by noise exposure starts in the dorsal cochlear nucleus. Changes of these types have also been identified in the inferior colliculus and cerebral cortex (the auditory cortex). From these findings we can now say that tinnitus certainly does involve several structures in the auditory system, not just one. 3) Imaging studies of human subjects with tinnitus have revealed areas of hyperactivation not only in the auditory system but also in the limbic system (see Chapter 3) of people who are bothered by their tinnitus. This was expected since for many years it has been known that the limbic system is involved in emotions, whether they're produced by sounds, thoughts or vision. 4) New studies are showing that tinnitus-related activity changes in the brainstem can be altered by stimulation of neurons outside the auditory system. For example, stimulation of nerve cells in the part of the nervous system dedicated to the sense of touch (the somatosensory system) can change the level of firing of neurons in the cochlear nucleus that are involved in tinnitus generation. This is important because many patients can alter their tinnitus percepts by certain manipulations, such as clenching of the jaws. This could lead to new ways of treating tinnitus that involve the somatosensory system, not just the auditory system.

**Step 2.** We've seen important progress made in developing measures of all these abnormalities and for measuring tinnitus. The degree of hyperactivity and bursting or synchronous firing that develop in the auditory systems of animals treated with tinnitus-inducing agents can now be measured routinely as part of the study of tinnitus. 2) It has been show in several studies that the same agents that cause animals to develop abnormal activity in their auditory systems also cause them to behave as if they have tinnitus. The demonstration of tinnitus-like percepts in animals is highly significant because this makes it much easier to study biological mechanisms that cause tinnitus (the goal of Path B). 3) Several methods have been developed for the measurement of "tinnitus" in animals. Methods for measuring tinnitus in human subjects have existed for many years, but they continue to become more refined, allowing characterization of tinnitus having different causes and features. A few studies have been able to predict from these measures what the tinnitus percepts (perceived sounds) produced by the abnormalities are likely to be. For example, in animal studies, when high activity is found in a given auditory brain center following noise exposure, it's typically found among neurons that respond best to high frequencies. This predicts that the tinnitus generated by this high activity would be high in pitch. We're now beginning to see some of the predictions receive support from measurements of the tinnitus sounds which animals experience after noise exposure.

**Step 3.** A growing number of studies are demonstrating that hyperactivity in the auditory system correlates with the presence of tinnitus. For example, hyperactivity in the dorsal cochlear nucleus (see Chapter 3) has been shown to be highest in animals with the strongest evidence of tinnitus and weakest in animals with the weakest evidence of tinnitus. This helps to bolster the case that increases in activity are an important cause of tinnitus.

## Path B Progress

**Step 1.** In the last decade, some important progress has been made in identifying the cell populations from which the tinnitus-related activity originates. In the dorsal cochlear nucleus, the cells that become hyperactive after noise exposure appear to include large neurons, called *fusiform cells.* These cells are likely to be important because they connect with higher levels of the auditory system, such as the inferior colliculus, which drives activity in the auditory cortex where conscious perceptions arise. This is to say: the hyperactivity of fusiform cells may be what drives the conscious perception of tinnitus. Similar studies need to be conducted at those higher levels to determine whether the tinnitus-producing activity is in fact channeled up along the pathway before it reaches the conscious level.

**Step 2.** Researchers are working to determine the chemical and anatomical defects that underlie tinnitus-related neural hyperactivity. It's now known that excessive noise exposure causes malfunction in the release of inhibitory transmitters, chemicals at the junctions between neurons, and this then fails to keep the postsynaptic cells quiet (see Chapter 3). Noise exposure also causes anatomical alterations in the number and structure of receptors for those transmitters. The receptors are the molecules on the cells that receive the neurotransmitters. They are the locks into which the neurotransmitter keys fit to change the activity of neurons. One of the main neurotransmitters affected is *glycine*. This is found throughout the brain and is known to play a role in the control of resting neural activity. The loss of glycine may be part of a more complex picture that includes breakdown and loss of inhibitory synapses—the connections between neurons. The theory that's emerging is that when these synapses are lost, the amount of glycine available for inhibiting resting activity is diminished, and this leads to an increase in resting activity or hyperactivity. Further increases in activity may arise because there are increases in the levels of excitatory synapses. There is evidence that noise exposure causes increases in the activity of excitatory synapses that use the neurotransmitters glutamate and acetylcholine. The increase in these synapses could further amplify the level of hyperactivity of affected neurons.

**Step 3.** It's becoming increasingly apparent that different forms of tinnitus may be triggered by different changes. As mentioned above, the type of tinnitus caused by excessive levels of aspirin seems to start in the inner ear. The active ingredient in aspirin (*salicylate*) blocks the functions of certain hair cells in the cochlea (see Chapter 7). The blockage of one type of hair cell (outer hair cells) causes increases in the activity of the auditory nerve. This type of tinnitus is usually reversible by ceasing use of aspirin. What about the chronic form of tinnitus? The most studied of these forms is noise-induced tinnitus. There's evidence that even this form of tinnitus is triggered by damage to the inner ear. We know that loss of outer hair cells can cause hyperactivity of neurons in the dorsal cochlear nucleus. A recent study points to degeneration of auditory nerve fibers as an important trigger of tinnitus. So we're beginning to see some significant progress in understanding the mechanisms underlying some defects that underlie tinnitus. But much remains to be done at other levels of the auditory system to determine which defect in which structures contribute the most to the generation of tinnitus signals.

### Path C Progress

**Step 1.** A large number of studies have been performed in Step 1 over the past decade. Some of the treatment modalities that have been tested so far include drug therapy, electrical stimulation, transcranial magnetic stimulation, surgical ablations or transections, sound therapy, or psychological counseling. The encouraging news is that most of the treatment modalities attempted have been reported to have some degree of benefit to at least some tinnitus patients. Sometimes the benefits have been remarkable for a few patients, but more typically, the benefits have been variable from one individual to the next, and are associated with undesirable side effects. Modalities that fit into this category are transcranial magnetic stimulation, electrical stimulation of the ear or auditory areas of the brain and most drug therapies. On the other hand, certain other treatment modalities that are non-invasive may have few or no side effects and may possibly have more benefit. A recent study of 35 patients using sound therapy reported an average 65% reduction in tinnitus disturbance after 6 months of use. A recent drug study indicated that nearly half of patients receiving Acamprosate (usually taken for alcohol addiction) reported an improvement of at least 50% in their tinnitus (see Chapter 11). Similar benefits have been reported for psychological counseling.

**Steps 2 and 3.** Progress is slowly being made in these steps, at least in dealing with the emotional reaction to tinnitus. There are many excellent treatments that use counseling and sound therapy. Both treatments are built on theory and knowledge arising from research in Paths A and B. Perhaps because counseling is guided by knowledge from psychology and of the pathways underlying emotional responses, counseling has proven to be highly effective in treating the emotional disturbance caused by tinnitus. You should be aware that the sounds of tinnitus may continue to be present, but the sound is no longer interpreted by the emotional centers of the brain as negative.

### Path D Progress

We're all waiting for developments in Path D, refining the treatments. Actually, there have been improvements in the counseling procedures (see Chapters 5, 6 and 9) as well as many new approaches in using sound therapy (Chapter 10). Certainly as drug, electrical and other treatments emerge, they'll be refined by contributions from other parts of the Roadmap.

## Tentative Conclusions of the Roadmap

We've learned a great deal about the processes in the ear and brain leading to tinnitus. But what we have is only a skeletal framework of understanding. We've been able to fill in some words in the crossword puzzle and some of these words are beginning to connect. But much more information is needed to complete the puzzle. When we understand the mechanism of tinnitus well enough, we'll be in a much better position to intervene and reverse the condition for each type of tinnitus without causing significant side effects. The roadmap, it is hoped, will help guide research toward the achievement of these goals.

Table 10-I: Tinnitus associations around the world

Action for Tinnitus Research
330-332 Gray's Inn Road
London, England
WC1X 8EE
020 7679 8907
www.tinnitus-research.org
help@tinnitus-research.org

American Tinnitus Association National Headquarters
PO Box 5
Portland, OR 97207-0005
(800) 634-8978 Toll Free within the United States
(503) 248-9985
(503) 248-0024 Fax
www.ata.org
tinnitus@ata.org

Australian Tinnitus Association
PO Box 660
Woollahra NSW 1350, Australia
(02) 8382-3331
(02) 8382-3333 Fax
www.tinnitus.asn.au
info@tinnitus.asn.au

(con't)

Better Hearing Australia Tinnitus Self Help Group
28 Gormanston Road,
Moonah Tasmania 7009, Australia
(03) 6228-0011

The British Tinnitus Association
Ground Floor, Unit 5
Acorn Business Park, Woodseats Close
Sheffield, S8 0TB, England
0800-018-0527
0114-258-2279 - Fax
www.tinnitus.org.uk
info@tinnitus.org.uk

French Tinnitus Association
France Acouphenes
73 rue Riquet
75018 Paris, France
01-42-05-01-46
04-67-48-94-37
www.france-acouphenes.org/la_revue/larevue.htm
aide-conseils@france-acouphenes.org

German Tinnitus League
Deutsche Tinnitus-Liga e.V. (DTL)
Postfach 210351
42353 Wuppertal, Germany
(0202) 24-65-2-0
(0202) 24-65-2-20 Fax
http://tinnitus-liga.de/index.php
dtl@tinnitus-liga.de

The Netherlands Tinnitus Association
Postbus 129, 3990 DC Houten, The Netherlands
(030) 261-76-16
(030) 261-66-89 Fax
(030) 261-76-77 Text Telephone
www.nvvs.nl
info@nvvs.nl

(con't)

Tinnitus Association of Canada
23 Ellis Park Rd
Toronto, ON M6S 2V4, Canada
(416)762-1490
www.kadis.com/ta/tinnitus.htm
elizabetheayrs@sympatico.ca

Tinnitus Association of Victoria
C/- Better Hearing Advisory Centre
5 High Street, Prahan Victoria 3181, Australia
(03) 9510-1577
(03) 9510-6076 Fax
www.tinnitusvic.asn.au
iap@alphalink.com.au

Tinnitus South Australia
51 Angas Street,
Adelaide 5000, Australia
1-300-789-988
www.tinnitussa.org
tinnitussa@chariot.net.au

## Tinnitus Glossary

**acamprosate** - a drug used for the treatment of alcohol dependence and recently applied to tinnitus treatment

**acoustic neuroma** - (also called vestibular schwannoma), benign (non-threatening) tumor typically originating from the balance branches of the combined hearing and balance nerve (the VIIIth Cranial Nerve)

**acoustic schwannoma** - benign tumor of the vestibular nerve

**acupuncture** - ancient Chinese practice of piercing parts of the body with needles in an effort to treat disease or relieve pain; has been applied to tinnitus treatment with no evidence of effectiveness

**adrenal cortex** - region of the brain that produces hormones related to stress and immune responses

**afferent** - (such as fibers) pertaining to the condition of the ascending nervous system tracts from peripheral to central (Ant: see *efferent*)

**Americans with Disabilities Act** - US law enacted to provide equal access for individuals with disabilities

**aminoglycoside antibiotics** - group of bacterial antibiotics which are often cochleotoxic and/or vestibulotoxic used commonly in streptomycin, neomycin, kanamycin and gentamicin

**amygdala** - region of the brain, located in the temporal lobe, believed to play a key role in the emotions, such as fear and pleasure and in memory

**anemia** - a condition in which there is a reduction in the number or volume of red blood corpuscles or of the total amount of hemoglobin (might be important for some forms of tinnitus)

**anesthetics** - a drug that causes partial or total loss of the sense of pain; some have been applied to tinnitus treatment with short-term results

**anticonvulsants** - drugs are primarily used to prevent seizures or control their incidence or severity and has been applied to tinnitus treatment

**antidepressants** - any drug or other substance used to treat depression (also see *tricyclic antidepressants*)

**artery lumen** - the small central space in an artery through which blood flows

**anxiety** - a state of worry, nervousness, tension and / or restlessness

**articulatory suppression** - a process of relaxation whereby you repeat a monosyllabic emotionally neutral word (such as "the") in a quiet or silent voice to yourself

**Attention Deficit Hyperactivity Disorder (ADHD)** - cognitive disorder involving reduced ability to focus on an activity, task or sensory stimulus, characterized by restlessness and distractibility, most common in children

**attenuate** - reduction in magnitude

**audiogram** - graphical representation of hearing from a hearing test

**audiologist** - healthcare practitioner who is credentialed in the practice of audiology to provide a comprehensive array of services related to prevention, evaluation and rehabilitation of hearing impairment, tinnitus and its associated communication disorder

**audiology** - branch of healthcare devoted to the study, diagnoses, treatment and prevention of hearing disorders, including tinnitus

**auditory cortex** - portion of the brain that it activated by sound, where the patterns of neural activity are combined to form words and sentences (in the temporal lobe)

**auditory habituation** - decline in the tendency to respond to sounds that have become familiar due to repeated exposure

**auditory nerve** - a bundle of nerve fibers that connects the synapses at the base of the inner hair cells to nerve fibers in the brainstem

**auditory system** - the entire system that processes sound, from the ear lobe through the cochlea to the auditory cortex

**autobiographical memory** - remembering a specific time and place, for example, "the day I lost my keys when cycling"

**autogenic relaxation** - a specific relaxation procedure involving visualizations while resting in relaxing positions (similar to meditation and yoga)

**axons** - long fibers that transmit messages from a cell body to other neurons

**basilar membrane** - located at the base of the membranous labyrinth of the cochlea, dividing it into the scala vestibule and scala tympani, that supports the scala media and organ of Corti

**benzodiazepines** - minor tranquilizers that act primarily upon the central nervous system and have a tranquillizer effect; promote sleep, muscle relaxation, have anticonvulsant properties and has been used in tinnitus treatment

**bilateral** - both sides

**biopsychosocial**- when the biology, psychology and social aspects of a situation are considered

**brainstem** - portion of the brain between the spinal cord and cerebrum (just below the brain)

**cardiovascular** - of the heart and the blood vessels as a unified body system

**central masking** - when one sound masks (covers up) another sound by processes in the brain

**cerebral insufficiency** - not enough blood reaching the brain, causing concentration difficulties, loss of memory, dizziness and perhaps tinnitus

**cerebral pontine angle** - a region of the brainstem, often a site for tumors

**cerumen** - earwax

**chemotherapy agents** - any drug typically taken for cancer treatment such as cisplatin

**cholesteatoma** - abnormal growth of skin behind the eardrum which forms a foul smelling pouch

**cilia** - hairs found at the top of the 'hair cells' in the cochlea; also in the vestibular (balance) end organ (see *cochlear hair cells*)

**cilium** - singular of cilia

**cochlea** - snail shaped bony capsule containing the end organ of hearing

**cochlear hair cells** - respond to movement and generate neural signals which are then sent via the auditory nerve and brainstem pathways up to the brain

**cochlear implant** - device that enables people with profound hearing loss to perceive sound, consisting of an electrode array surgically implanted in the cochlea that delivers electrical signals to the auditory cranial nerve

**cochlear nucleus** - cluster of cell bodies of second-order neurons on the lateral edge of the hindbrain in the central auditory nervous system at which fibers from Cranial Nerve VIII have an obligatory synapse

**cochleotoxic** - potential damage to the structures of the cochlea

**cognitive behavioral therapy (CBT)** - a formal psychotherapy that challenges thoughts about problems and practices behaviors to help change thoughts and reactions

**cognitive bias** - a tendency to selectively remember certain things more clearly and other things less clearly

**combination instruments** - refers to the use of a hearing aid with a built-in tinnitus masker

**compression limiting** - method of limiting maximum output of a hearing aid by means of compression circuitry

**conductive hearing loss** - reduction in hearing sensitivity, despite normal cochlear function, due to impaired sound transmission through the ear canal, eardrum or middle ear

**congenital** - from birth

**corticosteroids** - any of the steroid hormones secreted by the adrenal cortex, involved in many functions in the body such as stress response, immune response and regulation of inflammation; synthetic drugs with corticosteroid-like effect have been applied to tinnitus treatment

**cross-talk** - when information on one channel (or nerve) leaks across and interacts (or interferes) with a second channel (or nerve)

**cutaneous-evoked tinnitus** - tinnitus that is produced by touch on the skin

**cutaneous stimulation** - touching

**decibel Hearing Level (dB HL)** - unit of sound intensity based on a logarithmic relationship; 0 dB HL is normal hearing for young adults

**dendrites** - short fibers that receive messages from other neurons and relay them to the cell body

**dentist** - person whose profession is care of teeth and surrounding soft tissue

**depression** - an emotional condition, characterized by feelings of low mood, hopelessness and fatigue

**diabetes mellitus** - high blood glucose levels due to inability to metabolize carbohydrates

**dietary supplement** - a product taken by mouth that contains an ingredient intended to supplement the diet

**diuretics** - drugs that increase the excretion of urine

**dorsal cochlear nucleus** - one part of the cochlear nucleus, the first neural station in the brainstem receiving neurons from the cochlea; it also receives input from other neural systems higher in the brainstem

**ear coning** - (also called ear candling), a purported method to remove ear canal wax which is ineffective and dangerous

**eardrum** - thin membranous vibrating tissue terminating the ear canal and forming the major portion of the lateral wall of the middle ear cavity

**efferent** - (such as fibers), pertains to the conduction of the descending nervous system tracts from central to peripheral Ant: see afferent)

**elaboration** - processing information and making links with other information, such as memories of names, places, time and various aspects that will ensure the information is located at the right place in memory

**electroencephalograph (EEG)** - instrument used to record electrical potentials of the brain from electrodes attached to the scalp

**encoding** - how we take in information from our senses

**endocrine gland** - glands that produce hormones; the main endocrine glands are the pituitary gland, the pancreas, the gonads, the thyroid gland and the adrenal glands

**endocrinologist** - practice of medicine specializing in the diagnosis and treatment of diseases of the endocrine gland and their hormones

**endolymph(atic)** - a fluid found in the scala media of the cochlea having a high potassium and low sodium concentration

**endolymphatic hydrops** - excessive accumulation of endolymph fluid pressure in part of the body, believed to be the underlying disorder in Ménière's disease

**ephaptic communication** - electrical crosstalk in a thinning neural membrane

**Eustachian tube** - passageway leading from the back of the throat to the middle ear; it normally opens with movement of the mouth and equalizes pressure

**excitatory** - tending to excite or stimulate

**exocytosis** - a process of neurotransmitter release at the bottom of hair cells in a specialized area where packets of neurotransmitters are stored

**fibromyalgia** - a chronic condition causing pain, stiffness, and tenderness of the muscles, tendons, and joints; cause is currently unknown

**Food and Drug Administration (FDA)** - a division of the US Government mainly responsible for monitoring the safety and effectiveness of prescribed medications or substances that are seeking approval to be prescribed medications

**frequency** - the number of times a repetitive event occurs in a specified time period; specifically related to sound, the number of periods occurring in 1 second expressed in Hertz (Hz) or cycles per second

**functional imaging** - image techniques that show the brain in activity

**fusiform cells** - cells that become hyperactive after noise exposure which appear to include large neurons in the dorsal cochlear nucleus

**GABA** - chemical in the brain found at many levels of the central auditory pathway, and with modulation may be related to tinnitus

**gaze-evoked tinnitus** - tinnitus that can be initiated by eye movement

**geniculate body** - the medial geniculate body is part of the brainstem and the auditory system between the inferior colliculus and the auditory cortex

**Ginkgo biloba** - world's oldest living tree species whose extracts from leaves have been used for medicinal purposes for at least 5000 years in China

**glomus jugulare tumor** - (also called paraganglioma tumor), a vascular anomaly or malformation originating from the jugular vein which can in fact erode the bones surrounding the middle ear; if one examines the ear canal and the eardrum with an otoscope or a microscope one can see the reddish hue of this vascular anomaly as it invades the middle ear; if a glomus tumor is the source of the vascular tinnitus it requires immediate medical and surgical attention

**habituation** - when something is repeated over and over again without consequence, the response diminishes (see *auditory habituation*)

**hair cells** - see *cochlear hair cells*

**hemorrhagic agents** - drugs that improve blood flow changing the red blood cell properties, such as pentoxifylline

**Hertz (Hz)** - unit of measure of frequency representing number of cycles per second

**homeopathy** - based on the theory that it's possible to stimulate the body's defense mechanisms by giving small dosages of substances that would produce the illness if given in larger doses; not proven useful for tinnitus

**homeostasis** - the tendency to maintain normal or internal stability in an organism by coordinated responses of the organ systems that automatically compensate for environmental changes

**hyperacusis** - when sounds that are perceived as loud by most people are perceived as very loud ("loudness" hyperacusis)

**hyperbaric oxygen therapy** - breathing pure oxygen in a special chamber for treatment; has been applied for tinnitus treatment with inadequate data to report effectiveness

**hypertension** - high blood pressure

**hyperthyroidism** - overproduction of hormones such that their levels in the blood are high

**hypnotics** - drugs used specifically for improving sleeping

**hypothyroidism** - insufficient hormone is produced, which is also a risk factor for high cholesterol levels

**immittance** - test of mobility of ear drum to determine fluid behind the eardrum, or middle ear test to record middle-ear muscle reflexes

**incus** - see *ossicles*

**inferior colliculus** - auditory nucleus of the midbrain

**inhibitory** - tending to inhibit or restrain

**innervation** - distribution of nerve fibers to a structure

**insomnia** - difficulty falling asleep

**internal dialogue** - when hearing has been impaired for a long time and you lose some of your abilities to guess and to fill in the gaps

**lateral lemniscus** - a tract of nerve fibers in the brain that carries information from the cochlear nucleus to different relays in the brainstem

**limbic system** - brain structures including the hippocampus and amygdala that support a variety of functions including emotion, behavior and long term memory

**lipid** - any of a group of organic compounds consisting of the fats and other substances of similar properties (insoluble in water, greasy to the touch)

**lipid levels** - levels of fats in the blood (some lipids can worsen blood circulation)

**lipoproteins** - any group of proteins combined with a lipid found in blood plasma or egg yolk

**long-term memory** - aspect of the information-processing function of the central nervous system that receives, modifies and stores information on a permanent basis for later retrieval

**Loudness Discomfort Level** - a test by which sound is perceived to be uncomfortably loud (usually done under earphones)

**malleus** - see *ossicles*

**masking** - as pertains to tinnitus, when an external noise covers up the sound of one's tinnitus (total masking) or only partly covers up the tinnitus (partial masking) so that the tinnitus is still heard but at a lower loudness (also see *central masking*)

**medial geniculate body** - see geniculate body

**melatonin** - a hormone produced by the pineal gland that helps regulate sleep; preliminary studies suggest it decreases sleep problems in people with tinnitus

**Ménière's disease** - ear disease characterized by fluctuating hearing loss, tinnitus and aural fullness or pressure

**meningiomas** - usually benign but sometimes malignant tumors of the brain

**meninges** - the membranes covering the brain and spinal cord

**meningitis** - bacterial or viral inflammation of the meninges which can cause significant auditory disorder due to suppurative labyrinthitis or inflammation of the lining of Cranial Nerve VIII

**metabolic disturbances** - disturbances in processes involved in providing energy and maintaining the functions of cells and systems throughout the body

**middle ear** - air-filled cavity behind the eardrum that contains the ossicles

**millisecond** - (abbrev: ms), one thousandth of a second

**millivolt** - one thousandth of a volt

**multiple sclerosis** - neurologic disorder of unknown cause; widespread disease may affect auditory pathway

**myelin sheath** - protective cover (myelin) over a neural fiber

**myelinated** - insulation that covers parts of the nerve, minimizing "cross-talk" between the individual nerve fibers

**myoclonus** - twitching of a muscle or group of muscles

**nerve fibers** - a length of a nerve that carries information along the nervous system

**neural pathways** - groups of nerve fibers that carry information to the next station in a coordinated fashion

**neurofibromatosis II** - brainstem or cerebellopontine angle tumors

**neurological** - having to do with the nervous system, its structure and diseases

**neurologist** - practice of medicine specializing in the diagnosis and treatment of diseases of the nervous system

**neuron** - basic unit of the nervous system consisting of an axon, cell body and dendrite

**neurosurgeon** - branch of surgery involving the brain and spinal cord

**neurotransmitters** - chemical agents released by a presynaptic cell upon excitation that cross the synapse and excite or inhibit the post-synaptic cell

**noise trauma** - damage to hearing from excessive noise, sometimes the term is reserved for exposure to a transient, high frequency sound

**notched audiogram** - area of greatest loss on an audiogram, typically with noise-induced hearing loss may be around 3000 Hz or 4000 Hz

**nutritionist** - expert on foods, vitamins and nutrients

**objective tinnitus** - tinnitus that can be heard by an examiner

**olivocochlear bundle** - part of the auditory tract in the brainstem, which is the first area to receive neurons from both sides

**organ of Corti** - organ of hearing in the cochlea

**ossicles** - three tiny bones of the middle ear: malleus, incus and stapes

**ossicular chain** - see *ossicles*

**otitis media** - infection of the middle ear that persists with pus discharge, potentially leading to middle ear damage and eardrum perforation

**otolaryngologist** - practice of medicine specializing in the diagnosis and treatment of diseases of the ear, nose and throat

**otologist** - practice of medicine specializing in the diagnosis and treatment of diseases of the ear

**otosclerosis** - abnormal bony growth in the middle ear, particularly around the footplate of the stapes bone

**ototoxic** - a chemical that is capable of damage to the ear or hearing and can cause tinnitus

**oval window** - allows transfer of energy into the otherwise bony capsule of the cochlea

**palatal myoclonus** - a sudden and involuntary contraction of the roof of the mouth muscles, which results in clicking or popping in the ear.

**paraganglioma tumor** - see: *glomus jugulare tumor*

**peak clipping** - process of restricting the maximum output of a hearing aid by limiting amplitude peaks at a fixed level

**pediatrician** - a physician whose practice specialty is the care of infants and children

**peripheral vascular disease** - insufficient blood flow to the limbs because of damage to blood vessels

**phantom limb** - the illusion that something is present when it isn't; for example, feeling of moving the fingers in an amputated hand

**pharmacological** - the science dealing with the effect of drugs on living organisms

**phase cancellation** - when two signals that are identical except opposite in phase (one moves a diaphragm inwards while at the same time the other moves a diaphragm outwards) are added together

**phase locking** - tendency of nerve fibers to fire at a particular phase of the stimulating waveform

**phonophobia** - an unrealistic fear of sound, sometimes called fear hyperacusis

**physiotherapist** - health professionals that assess patients and plan and carry out individually designed treatment programs to maintain, improve or restore physical functioning, alleviate pain and prevent physical dysfunction in patients.

**pinna** - outer cartilaginous portion of the ear

**plasticity** - ability of the brain to change and adapt

**post-masking relief** - another term for residual inhibition

**post-traumatic stress disorder (PTSD)** - a condition characterized by recurring and often disabling symptoms of anxiety and depression originating from a traumatic event

**presbycusis** - hearing loss due to aging

**progressive muscle relaxation exercises** - a mixture of physical tensing/relaxing techniques, breathing exercises and mental imagery to reduce tension, agitation and arousal

**psychiatrist** - branch of medicine specializing in treatment and prevention of disorders of the mind

**psychosocial** - pertaining to the psychological development of the individual in relation to his or her social environment

**pulsatile tinnitus** - a sound like blood vessels pulsing

**rapid eye movements (REMs)** - brief periods during deep sleep when the eyes move very quickly

**recruitment** - abnormal loudness growth of sound as the intensity is increased in a sensorineural-impaired ear

**refractory period** - the time it takes for an auditory nerve fiber to recuperate before it can fire again

**relaxation exercises** - see progressive muscular relaxation

**residual inhibition** - when tinnitus actually disappears for a period of time following some external stimulus stopping, such as a masking device being turned off

**retrieval** - when information is retrieved from memory or when we make use of stored information in the brain

**rheumatologist** - practice of medicine specializing in diagnosis and treatment of rheumatic diseases (painful condition of the joints and muscles)

**ribbon synapse** - the bottom of the hair cells are specialized areas where packets of neurotransmitters are stored, tethered or attached to a ribbon-like structure that forms a pool of packets waiting to be released

**salicylate** - a salt of salicylic acid commonly found in aspirin

**selective attention** - highly focused attention at the exclusion of other events; a person who believes that tinnitus is a threat to well-being will focus attention on tinnitus to the exclusion of other things

**selective serotonin reuptake inhibitors** - prevents re-absorption of serotonin, one of the brain chemicals thought to cause depression

**sensorineural hearing loss** - cochlear or retrocochlear loss in hearing

**serotonin** - a neurotransmitter and hormone found in the blood that constricts the blood vessels and contracts smooth muscle tissue

**short-term memory** - aspect of the information-processing function of the central nervous system that receives, modifies, stores information briefly

**sign language** - form of manual communication in which words and concepts are represented by hand positions and movements

**somatosensory** - broad term relating to the sensory systems that are responsible for touch (and pressure), pain, movement, position of body parts and temperature

**speechreading** - the process of visual recognition of speech communication, combining lipreading with observation of facial expressions and gestures

**stapedectomy** - an operation whereby the stapes bone is separated from the incus and the bony growth around the oval window is cleared away, then a prosthesis is connected to the incus and sealed around the oval window, replacing the function of the stapes bone, and restoring hearing

**stapedius muscle** - one of two striated muscles (also see *tensor tympani*) in the middle ear innervated by the facial nerve

**stapes** - see *ossicles*

**subcortical** - areas below the cortex often implying in the brainstem, at the base of the brain

**subjective tinnitus** - tinnitus that cannot be heard by the examiner

**successive approximations** - a desensitization procedure used in treatment of some phobias for the purpose of adaptation, a technique also applied in treatment of hyperacusis

**sudden idiopathic sensorineural hearing loss** - rapid onset of hearing loss, typically unilateral, usually substantial with unknown causes and uncertain prognosis for recovery

**superior olivary complex** - collection of auditory nuclei in the hindbrain that relay information from the cochlear nucleus to the midbrain

**synapse** - activity of one nerve fiber passed on to another at neural junctions

**syphilis** - venereal disease caused by a bacteria and usually transmitted by sexual intercourse or acquired congenitally

**tea** - dried and prepared leaves used to make a beverage; for tinnitus the herbal extracts have been used for their sedative qualities (unproven)

**tectorial membrane** - membrane within the cochlea in which cilia of the outer hair cells are embedded

**temporal lobe** - portion of the cerebrum that houses the primary auditory cortex

**temporomandibular joint (TMJ)** - point of articulation between the mandible and temporal bone

**tensor tympani** - one of two striated muscles (also see *stapedius*) in the middle ear innervated by the trigeminal nerve

**tinnitus** - (also see *objective* and *subjective*), sensation of ringing, buzzing, whooshing or other sound in the ears or head without an external stimulus

**tinnitus masker** - a device used to produce a sound to partially or totally mask the tinnitus,(also see *masking*)

**tonotopic map** - an orderly array that is organized according to frequency

**transcranial magnetic stimulation** - a non-invasive (no surgery or implant is needed) procedure that generates a changing magnetic field across the skull and influences brain activity

**transduction process** - when hair cells are stimulated so that mechanical movements of the cochlea are converted to electrical action potentials in the nerve

**tricyclic antidepressants** - block the re-absorption of certain chemicals in the brain and present antidepressant and analgesic effects

**tympanic membrane** - term for the eardrum

**tympanosclerosis** - scarring of the eardrum caused by previous inflammation or infection, leading to hearing loss

**unilateral** - pertaining to one side only

**valerian root** - an herb used to help people sleep

**vasodilators** - anything that causes widening of the blood vessels (such drugs as betahistine or the natural Chinese herb ginkgo biloba)

**vascular loop** - intracranial blood vessels that happen to loop and coil around the balance part of the VIIIth Cranial Nerve (the one responsible for hearing too, in the brainstem)

**vestibulotoxic** - potential damage to the vestibule of the inner ear

**vitamins** - compounds required for essential reactions in the body and for normal growth, development, maintenance of cells, tissues and organs

**whiplash** - sudden flexion and extension movement of the cervical spine caused by car accidents

**white noise** - broadband noise having equal energy at all frequencies

**working memory** - area of the brain (not completely identified) used to store and process information

**zinc** - a mineral present in all organs, tissues, fluids and secretions of the body, and essential to human body function; its deficiency might be related to tinnitus

Compiled in part from: Stach, BA. Comprehensive Dictionary of Audiology. (1997). Baltimore: Williams & Wilkins Co; and Webster's New World Dictionary. (1994). Third College Ed., NY: Prentice-Hall.

# B

# C

# I

# W

# Z

## NOTES

NOTES